The daily practices that Judith offers sing of her honesty, compassion, and wisdom. She knows just where the pitfalls are and how to wake us up to the teacher within, to live each moment from our authentic source. Like a koan, these often humorous and surprising sayings can help reveal and shape a life of fresh relationship: to yoga, to ourselves, and to the world.

—*Jiko Linda Ruth Cutts, Abbess;*
*Green Gulch Farm, San Francisco Zen Center*

Judith is eloquent and can expound upon the lofty idealism of yoga better than almost anyone. But her forte is truly in her commitment to finding ways to actualize its teachings into a seamless experience in which life and yoga are not separate. This book is meant to be used by all who wish to bring yoga to life!

—*Sharon Gannon, coauthor*
*(with David Life) of* Jivamukti Yoga

One thread, one sutra at a time, Judith Hanson Lasater weaves together mindfulness, daily life, meditation, yoga, the sacred, and the profane. This essential book—a luminous tapestry—enables life and yoga to become one again.

—*François Raoult, M.A., director of*
*Open Sky Yoga Center, Rochester, New York*

Judith's words of wisdom have inspired me since I took my first workshop with her in the early 1970s. Every time we meet, whether at a yoga conference or for tea, I am uplifted by her even outlook on things. I can't wait to experience a year guided by her daily measure of insight into the workings of the human mind and body.

— *Beryl Bender Birch, author of* Power Yoga

This book will inspire you to live your yoga—all day, every day. With wisdom and clarity, Judith offers 365 opportunities to embrace the ordinary as sacred. Who knew that fresh sheets, driving the speed limit, growing old, and juicy apples could be the path to an awakened life!

— *Cyndi Lee, author of* Yoga Body, Buddha Mind

# A YEAR OF
# LIVING YOUR YOGA

By Judith Hanson Lasater, Ph.D., P.T.

*Relax and Renew* (1995)

*Living Your Yoga* (2000)

*30 Essential Yoga Poses* (2003)

*Yoga for Pregnancy* (2004)

*Yoga Abs* (2005)

*A Year of Living Your Yoga* (2006)

# A YEAR
# OF LIVING
# YOUR YOGA

## DAILY PRACTICES
## TO SHAPE YOUR LIFE

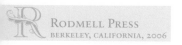

RODMELL PRESS
BERKELEY, CALIFORNIA, 2006

Judith Hanson Lasater, Ph.D., P.T.

*A Year of Living Your Yoga: Daily Practices to Shape Your Life,*
copyright © 2006 by Judith Hanson Lasater, Ph.D., P.T. All rights reserved.

Library of Congress Cataloging-in-Publication Data
Lasater, Judith.
  A year of living your yoga : daily practices to shape your life /
Judith Hanson Lasater. — 1st ed.
     p. cm.
  ISBN-13: 978-1-930485-15-0 (alk. paper)
  ISBN-10: 1-930485-15-8 (alk. paper)
  1. Yoga—Quotations, maxims, etc. 2. Lasater, Judith—
Quotations.  I. Title.
B132.Y6L34 2006
181'.45—dc22                                           2006015204


First edition
13  12       6  7  8

ISBN 13: 978-1-930485-15-0

Editor: Linda Cogozzo
Associate Editor: Holly Hammond
Cover and Text Design: Gopa & Ted2, Inc.
Printed in China by Kwong Fat Offset Printing Co., Ltd.

Text set in Sabon • Distributed by Publishers Group West

# CONTENTS

# ACKNOWLEDGMENTS

THE PROCESS OF writing a book is not new to me. Nevertheless, it remains exciting and fulfilling. This is due, in part, to the help I receive from many sources.

My inspiration for *A Year of Living Your Yoga* was our first son, Miles. When he joined our life, I had a powerful reason to learn more about love, giving, and letting go. Throughout the years, he and his siblings, Kam and Elizabeth, have been my greatest gifts. I am grateful and full.

I appreciate those who contributed to the book that you hold in your hands:

My husband, Ike, who helped me to clarify my thinking and writing;

Sally and David Elsberry, my first yoga teachers, and Sri B. K. S. Iyengar, whose fiery teaching has helped me refine my practice throughout the years.

Kathy Vasquez, a yoga teacher in Anchorage, Alaska, who attends my annual retreats at Feathered Pipe Ranch in Helena,

Montana, and wrote down the aphorisms that are collected herein;

Beryl Bender Birch, Jiko Linda Ruth Cutts, Sharon Gannon, Cyndi Lee, and François Raoult, my friends and colleagues, for their generous words of praise;

The team at Rodmell Press, for their vision and expertise: Linda Cogozzo, editor; Holly Hammond, associate editor; and Gopa and Veetam Campbell, book and cover designers at Gopa & Ted2, Inc.

Donald Moyer and Linda Cogozzo, my publishers at Rodmell Press, for their help and support;

And my students, who have taught me not only how to teach, but also how to live more fully from my heart.

# PREFACE

I BEGAN MY YOGA STUDIES with Judith Hanson Lasater in the summer of 1976, at Feathered Pipe Ranch in Helena, Montana. I had been living in Alaska, so I had no access to teacher training, and I was hungry for information. Back then the teaching format at the Pipe was two teachers, two groups, and two different classes each morning and afternoon. In the morning, I would take Judith's two-and-a-half-hour asana class, where I gathered experiential knowledge of asana. In the afternoon, I would sit in the gallery above the yoga room and observe Judith as she taught. I took notes about what she did, how she did it, and the words she said—verbatim.

From the asana classes, I learned about alignment and how to invite yoga into the very tissues of my body. Observing Judith in the second class gave me a different vantage point, literally and figuratively. Watching her teach was (and still is) like witnessing a ballet: artful, fluid, with a perfect balance between energy and stillness, movement and pause.

From observing her teach, I have understood the importance of words, touch, stories, demonstration, and laughter. Her images evoke responses in the body that lead to alignment; her words inspire the heart to open wide and let in the truth. I watched this happen time and again, not only for me but for an entire room full of people, summer after summer. Judith has a deep respect for the power of words, so her teaching is extraordinarily clear. I am blessed that she teaches the way I learn. I don't have to struggle for the information. Each class becomes a dance in effortless effort.

I never tire of gathering information and inspiration from Judith's classes. Thirty years later I am still the scribe in the corner, taking down every word. Writing the words is another level of imprinting them, and this process has served me well throughout my yoga journey.

I am often asked whether I read those hundreds of pages after I return from a workshop with Judith. I always say there is too much gold there not to revisit those memorable moments—both for myself and for my students.

In 2002 I was delighted when Judith asked me to send her the aphorisms I had recorded, explaining that they were to be used in this book. I retrieved my notebooks from my basement yoga archives and spent two hours each Sunday afternoon reminiscing and compiling quotes from 1976 to the present. I feel such deep gratitude for the opportunity to record them the first time around and for the joy they evoked in me this time through. I was struck by the truth that still shines through her words.

Judith's words are with me in every yoga class I teach. I am currently enjoying the aphorism I wrote down in March 2006: "Life isn't lived through information. Stand in your truth and teach from your heart." Thank you, Judith, for your friendship and for sharing your extraordinary gifts with us.

—Kathy Vasquez
Anchorage, Alaska, 2006

*Yoga is the willingness to be present.*
—Judith Hanson Lasater, Ph.D., P.T.

# INTRODUCTION

TODAY, YOGA IS EQUATED with the practice of *asana* (yoga poses). However, asana is only part of a larger philosophy that includes other practices like *pranayama* (breathing) and *dhyana* (meditation). Even deeper than these practices is yoga's philosophy that teaches the transformative possibilities of awareness. Being in this state of awareness, or presence, helps us to live more fully, with less suffering and with more happiness.

How do you take the awareness that you cultivate on your yoga mat and meditation cushion into what you do all day long? Is it even possible? I think it is. You can begin by paying attention to the small things: circumstance by circumstance, moment by moment, and breath by breath. As you do, you will discover that awareness of the ordinary and mundane can enliven your on-the-mat practices. And then a new territory opens before you, in which life and practice are seamless. *A Year of Living Your Yoga* is designed to support your exploration—one day at a time, over the course of a year.

This book grew out of *Living Your Yoga,* which I wrote in 2000. In the first book, I wrote essays that centered around themes like love, patience, control, and spiritual seeking. I connected yoga philosophy to daily life by recounting anecdotes from my life, weaving in inspiration from the Yoga Sutra and the Bhagavad Gita. I rounded out each chapter with simple practices and Mantras for Daily Living. My intention was to help you see all of life as practice. The reader response has been so tremendous that I decided to take the idea of life as practice even further.

In *A Year of Living Your Yoga,* I present an aphorism, or teaching, for each day, plus how to practice by carrying the intention of the aphorism throughout your day. How the aphorisms came to be collected in this book is an interesting story in itself, as told in the preface by Kathy Vazquez, a yoga teacher from Anchorage, Alaska.

The aphorisms and practices cluster around themes such as cultivating attention, enjoying life, observing the mind, practicing from love, finding yourself, letting go of self-judgment, and more. The variety of practices will help you to see yourself, your life, and your practice in a new light. There is a mix of practices, such as asana, Mantras for Daily Living, noting, breathing, Savasana (Basic Relaxation Pose), and writing.

The book follows the calendar year. You can start with today's date. Begin by reflecting on the aphorism and then take up the practice. When is the best time? Here are some suggestions:

- upon awakening
- while having a cup of tea each morning
- just before stepping on your yoga mat
- sitting on your yoga mat a few minutes before doing asana
- before lying down to practice Savasana (Basic Relaxation Pose)
- on the train to or from work
- on your lunch break
- sitting in your garden

Here are some other suggestions for using the book:

- reread the day's entry and reflect on your practice of it before you fall asleep
- write about your practice experiences in your journal
- if you miss one or more days, just pick up from today
- on special days, such as your birthday, or an anniversary of a special event in your life, or a holiday, do something nurturing for yourself that includes *A Year of Living Your Yoga*
- find yourself a practice buddy to check in with once a week about how bringing yoga to life is going for each of you
- start the book again when you complete your first year

If you are a yoga teacher, consider using the book in these ways:

- read an aphorism and practice to your class just before Savasana (Basic Relaxation Pose)

- form a study group to discuss the practices with your students and other teachers
- use it in your teacher training program

Whatever you decide, I invite you to use *A Year of Living Your Yoga* in any way you like. Be flexible: your needs two months from now may be different than they are today.

My intention is to support and inspire you to embrace the limitless possibilities of yoga. Live it!

*To Miles Hanson Lasater,*
*who has taught me about living my yoga*
*every day since he was born.*

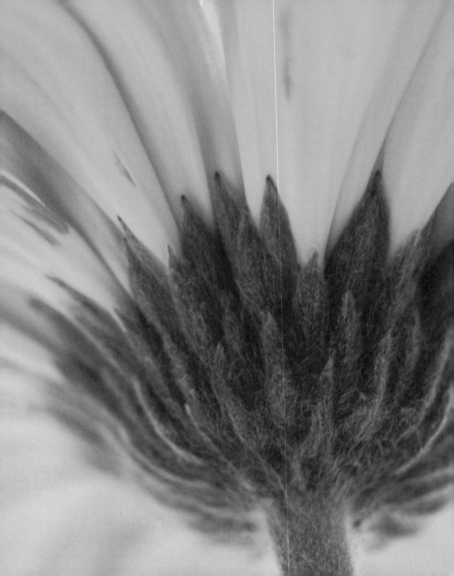

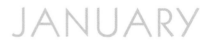

JANUARY

## JANUARY 1

*Living well is not about being calm; it is about being present.*

**LIVING YOUR YOGA:** For five minutes today, practice just being present with your emotions without reacting to them. Notice how they come and go.

## JANUARY 2

*Relaxation is the process of observing your tension.*

**LIVING YOUR YOGA:** Find a quiet place. Lie down on a comfortable surface, close your eyes, and observe your tension for ten minutes. Relaxation will arise.

## JANUARY 3

*We are not seeing a situation as it truly is if we have expectations.*

**LIVING YOUR YOGA:** The next time you are involved in a conflict, notice how you want things to turn out your way. Ask yourself, *How would this be and what would I say now if I could see what the other person sees?*

## JANUARY 4
*Laugh more.*

LIVING YOUR YOGA: Children laugh dozens of times a day. Laughing decreases blood pressure and relieves tension. Find something funny in your life today and laugh at it. Better yet, find something about yourself to laugh at.

## JANUARY 5
*Do what you love.*

LIVING YOUR YOGA: Doing what you love is empowering and even health-enhancing. Pick something, such as listening to your favorite piece of music, planting some flowers, or petting your dog, and do it for ten minutes today—just because you love it.

## JANUARY 6
*Trust yourself first.*

LIVING YOUR YOGA: Others can offer us advice and help, but deep inside we always know what is best for us. Today consciously choose to trust yourself first when you make a decision.

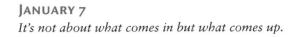

## JANUARY 7
*It's not about what comes in but what comes up.*

LIVING YOUR YOGA: We often believe that what we learn from the outside makes us better yoga students. Today when you practice, pay more attention to your own wisdom as it comes up.

## JANUARY 8
*Never throw away your filter.*

LIVING YOUR YOGA: Despite the wisdom and power of the teacher, you are the only master of yourself. Listen with a loving filter to your teacher, then absorb what resonates and let go of what doesn't.

## JANUARY 9
*Thinking is active; awareness is receptive.*

LIVING YOUR YOGA: Sit quietly in a comfortable position for five minutes, and let yourself just receive each moment as it arises. No thinking, no judgments.

## JANUARY 10

*We don't injure what we respect.*

**LIVING YOUR YOGA:** Treat all people you meet and all objects you handle with respect. At the end of the day, notice how happy you feel.

## JANUARY 11

*Practicing yoga is a loving act of respect.*

**LIVING YOUR YOGA:** In your practice today, treat your body with the respect you would give to my body.

## JANUARY 12

*Yoga practice allows our suffering to come to the surface.*

**LIVING YOUR YOGA:** Practice one of your favorite asana. When you feel the stretch, hold the pose, breathe, and let the stretch resolve itself.

## JANUARY 13

*Honor yourself as part of the Infinite.*

**LIVING YOUR YOGA:** Once today, close your eyes, and imagine that you are part of all that is around you, regardless of whether you like it or not.

## JANUARY 14
*With what attitude do you challenge your body?*

LIVING YOUR YOGA: In order find balance between the need to challenge yourself and the need to nurture yourself, choose this Mantra for Daily Living when you practice asana today: *I will move at the speed of my body, not my brain.*

## JANUARY 15
*Feel what you are feeling.*

LIVING YOUR YOGA: Sit down for a moment, close your eyes, and just feel what you are feeling: be with anger, with happiness, with boredom, or with fatigue. Do not judge this feeling. As you watch them, notice how your feelings transform.

## JANUARY 16
*Yoga does not solve our problems.*

LIVING YOUR YOGA: One of the greatest sources of our suffering is the attachment we have to finding "the solution." Right now practice Adho Mukha Svanasana (Downward-Facing Dog Pose) for itself, not because it stretches your hamstrings or shoulders. Breathe and enjoy it right now.

## JANUARY 17

*Problems are transformed when we are present.*

LIVING YOUR YOGA: When someone disagrees with you today, stay present, listen, and then let them solve the problem.

## JANUARY 18

*Yoga is the willingness to be present.*

LIVING YOUR YOGA: You can practice yoga all day, not just on your mat. How? When you are truly present, you are practicing yoga. Throughout your day, repeat this Mantra for Daily Living: *Right here, right now.*

## JANUARY 19

*Suffering comes from our unwillingness to be present.*

LIVING YOUR YOGA: Today notice five recurring thoughts that take you away from your life as it is. Write them down. When you have a chance, burn the paper lovingly, and let those thoughts drift away with the smoke.

## JANUARY 20
*Yoga practice allows the pain that is already in us*
*to be experienced.*

LIVING YOUR YOGA: When you practice your poses today, do not think of the gentle discomfort you feel as a problem. Remember that the tightness in your muscles is just your suffering trying to get out.


## JANUARY 21
*Be with what is.*

LIVING YOUR YOGA: Look out your window right now and see what is there: a perfectly manicured lawn, a busy sidewalk, an old shed falling down. Breathe it in.


## JANUARY 22
*A yoga practitioner is one who neither runs from*
*nor seeks out pain.*

LIVING YOUR YOGA: If your usual yoga practice is strong and stimulating, today try restorative yoga poses instead. If your practice is gentle, today do five of your hardest poses. Cultivate a nonjudging mind while you do them.

## JANUARY 23

*Work in a way that does not create more stress.*

**LIVING YOUR YOGA:** Work is necessary but making it stressful is not. When you go to work today, breathe before you answer the phone and pause for one breath before you answer your boss.

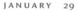

## JANUARY 24

*We spend too much time trying to fix everything.*

**LIVING YOUR YOGA:** Write down the three most common thoughts you have about how you should fix yourself and others. Remember, trying to fix yourself and others never really works. Instead, revel in your individuality and celebrate the uniqueness of others.

## JANUARY 25

*Be who you are, where you are.*

**LIVING YOUR YOGA:** The more we are ourselves, the more we enjoy our life. Today if you are in an uncomfortable, even restrictive situation, don't be afraid to speak your truth with love.

## JANUARY 26

*Without discipline there is no art.*

**LIVING YOUR YOGA:** The art of yoga comes from the consistency of discipline. Today resolve to practice for the next twenty-one days without missing a single one. Note it on your calendar.

## JANUARY 27

*Discipline arises from clarity of intention and commitment.*

**LIVING YOUR YOGA:** Sit quietly on your mat. Create an intention for your practice before you begin, such as this Mantra for Daily Living: *Today I will focus my practice on inviting inner stillness.*

## JANUARY 28

*Feeling at ease does not mean feeling nothing.*

**LIVING YOUR YOGA:** Three times today, stop, close your eyes, and ask yourself, *What am I feeling right now? Can I be at ease with it?* Name it and wait for the answer.

## JANUARY 29

*Why do we resist life?*

LIVING YOUR YOGA: When you feel resistance arising, first notice it. With a curious mind, allow yourself to acknowledge completely the aspect of your life that your resistance represents.


## JANUARY 30

*Every asana is about opening.*

LIVING YOUR YOGA: Today when you practice, find a new part of your body that is opening in each asana, even during a forward bend that seems to be about closing.


## JANUARY 31

*Yoga is not about avoiding difficulty.*

LIVING YOUR YOGA: When we try to avoid difficulty, we create difficulty. Today choose something you find difficult and do it with love for five minutes.

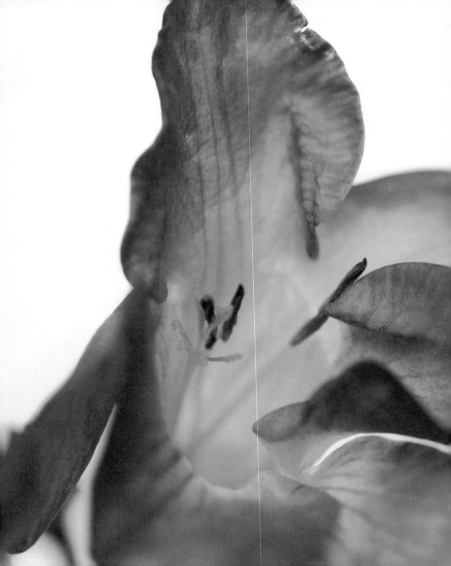

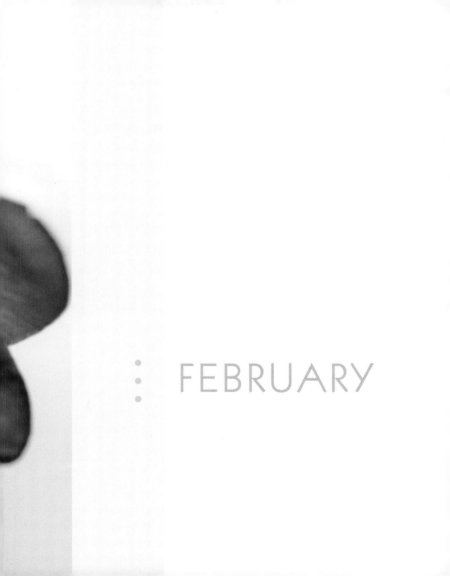

FEBRUARY

## FEBRUARY 1

*The goal of yoga is adaptability, not flexibility.*

LIVING YOUR YOGA: Many students come to asana practice in order to become more flexible. More important is learning to be adaptable and to let life flow through you. How can you do this in your practice today?

## FEBRUARY 2

*Each moment has the same potential for wholeness.*

LIVING YOUR YOGA: Wholeness is found not only in the special moments of being lost in an exquisite sunset or feeling the perfect balance of stillness in meditation. Every moment of your life can be just as whole if you allow it to be so. Today find the treasure in the most mundane moments. How did it go?

## FEBRUARY 3

*Life is holy.*

LIVING YOUR YOGA: One of my favorite verses of the Yoga Sutra of Patanjali (I:23) can be expressed as *Practice the presence of God.* Can you find God in the ritual of a forward bend or the softness of an inhalation done with awareness? When you do this, God becomes a practice, not just an idea.

## FEBRUARY 4

*Become a larger container for Spirit.*

**LIVING YOUR YOGA:** Recently, a friend recounted to me a situation in which she experienced what she called the "shocking pettiness" of her life. As you practice today, imagine yourself with a bigger heart, and from there bestow your generosity. For example, give away something to a person who needs it, or better yet give your long-overdue forgiveness.


## FEBRUARY 5

*The depth of my practice is revealed by how many times a day I get angry.*

**LIVING YOUR YOGA:** We cannot become angry unless we believe we are right. Today when you feel irritated about something, breathe deeply and allow being right to melt into being present.


## FEBRUARY 6

*Practice is uncovering the resistance.*

**LIVING YOUR YOGA:** Step on your mat and practice Adha Mukha Svanasana (Downward-Facing Dog Pose). Breathe into your physically tight spots and into your mental agitation. Remember that practice allows resistance to surface so it can fly away.

## FEBRUARY 7

*Everyone has to go through the woods and meet the Big Bad Wolf in order to get to Grandma's house.*

LIVING YOUR YOGA: We grow up when we realize no one's life is perfect or easy. Spend a quiet moment and take stock of your blessings. Say aloud, *Today I am grateful for ___.* Then realize that, even with problems, on the deepest level your life is perfect.

## FEBRUARY 8

*Impatience is the surface of anger.*

LIVING YOUR YOGA: Anger takes many forms. Count how many times today you feel frustrated, or irritated, or impatient. These are the number of times you have disconnected from yourself.

## FEBRUARY 9

*People who do not occasionally fall on their faces are not growing.*

LIVING YOUR YOGA: Try something that you cannot do at all, such as skateboarding, speaking the Sanskrit names of asana, or just thinking a radically new thought. Today failure is irrelevant.

## FEBRUARY 10

*Ninety-five percent of the mind is unconscious.*

LIVING YOUR YOGA: Remember that what you think is not all that you know. Consciously exhale and invite yourself to be comfortable with not knowing enough. No one does: not about ourselves, not about teaching yoga, not about the world.

## FEBRUARY 11

*I will be happy when I ___.*

LIVING YOUR YOGA: No accomplishment alone provides happiness. Consciously inhale, and as you exhale hold in your heart–mind someone or something that stimulates feelings of happiness within you. Keep this image for five long, easy breaths. Happiness is now.

## FEBRUARY 12

*Whatever you do, do it with an open heart.*

LIVING YOUR YOGA: Maybe you agreed to do something but now you are wishing you hadn't. If you do choose to follow through in the end, do so with willingness and interest. You will suffer less and so will the others around you.

## FEBRUARY 13
*When I am resisting, I am suffering.*

LIVING YOUR YOGA: Resisting life is the root of all suffering. If you feel agitated, sad, or afraid today, ask yourself, *What am I resisting?*

## FEBRUARY 14
*Observing weakens resistance.*

LIVING YOUR YOGA: Fighting with something makes it stronger. Today when you want to push something away, instead just sit down, close your eyes, and for five minutes imagine yourself as a large container holding your own resistance. The resistance may remain but you are fighting it no longer. This is freedom.

## FEBRUARY 15
*The more difficult a thing is, the more it requires softness.*

LIVING YOUR YOGA: When we encounter a difficult person, or situation, or asana, we often respond with hardness. In your practice today, choose a difficult pose and approach it with both mental and physical softness. Become like the water that flows around a rough boulder, gently washing against its edges.

## FEBRUARY 16

*We are seeking wholeness, not perfection.*

**LIVING YOUR YOGA:** Find a wood floor and spend a minute looking at what could be called its imperfections, such as knots, irregular grain, and discolorations. Remember that these imperfections are what give the floor its beauty and character; they make it real. Allow yourself to grow in wholeness, imperfections and all.

## FEBRUARY 17

*The breath is the gateway to consciousness.*

**LIVING YOUR YOGA:** Sit on a carpeted floor in a quiet room. Lie on a blanket that is 3 inches thick and 6 inches wide, and that you have positioned from your sacrum to your head. Then place another blanket under your head, and cover your eyes with a face cloth. Gently separate your arms away from your torso and your legs away from each other. Breathe in and out slowly twenty times. Then roll to the side, sit up, and notice your inner state.

## FEBRUARY 18
*Whatever you do, you will regret.*

LIVING YOUR YOGA: No matter how wonderful a decision you make, you will at another moment regret it. No matter how happily married or deeply grateful for your child you may be, for a few seconds, once in a while, you will regret your decision to marry or have a child. Resolve now that when that happens, you will embrace this fleeting sense of regret as a sign of your deep humanness and move on.

## FEBRUARY 19
*There is negative and positive in every situation.*

LIVING YOUR YOGA: Wisdom comes from seeing that all choices have pluses and minuses. Let this be today's Mantra for Daily Living. Repeat it to yourself and smile when you do so.

## FEBRUARY 20
*When we are happy and loving, we automatically find God.*

LIVING YOUR YOGA: Notice when you are happy today, and imagine following that happiness. Maybe it comes when singing a song with your child or practicing an asana you love. These moments are the door home to God.

## FEBRUARY 21
*Wherever your heart leads, follow.*

LIVING YOUR YOGA: Which would you rather live with, the mistakes of following your head or the mistakes of following your heart? Without throwing out common sense, today listen a little more to your heart whenever you can, and notice how satisfying your day becomes.


## FEBRUARY 22
*Your innate state is already holy.*

LIVING YOUR YOGA: If we practice because we feel not good enough, then practice can become another form of punishment. Today as you get on your yoga mat, say, *I am already holy*. Abide in the understanding that your practice expresses this truth with each breath.


## FEBRUARY 23
*Insecurity leads to more attempts to control.*

LIVING YOUR YOGA: We feel insecure when we forget our connection to ourselves. Then we feel afraid and try to control everything around us. Instead, spend five minutes today sitting quietly, focusing on elongating your exhalation; it is the breath of letting go.

## FEBRUARY 24
*There is nothing wrong with you.*

LIVING YOUR YOGA: Remember that although you may have problems, you are not a problem. At your core, you are whole and healthy. Offer this understanding to yourself at least three times today.


## FEBRUARY 25
*The greatest discipline is surrender.*

LIVING YOUR YOGA: So often we confuse ambition with discipline. We think pushing ourselves to do more proves we are disciplined. When you practice asana today, focus instead on how much clarity and discipline is required to let go: of your expectations, of yesterday's asana, of what may no longer be possible for you, of your resistance to doing what is possible.


## FEBRUARY 26
*Separateness is a false perception.*

LIVING YOUR YOGA: When we feel separate from ourselves, others, or the Universe, we suffer. Scientists and sages tell us that we are all *literally* interconnected. Today spend some quiet time remembering a moment of profound connection in your life. Be grateful for it.

## FEBRUARY 27

*If you want to embrace the light, you must also embrace the darkness.*

**LIVING YOUR YOGA:** We all long for love, peace, and ease. But in order to fully experience them, we must also be willing to embrace our hatred, anger, and agitation. Today when you feel any strong negative emotions, really feel them. Cutting off negative feelings cuts off our ability to feel all emotions.

## FEBRUARY 28

*Embrace your humanness first so that you can then embrace your Divinity.*

**LIVING YOUR YOGA:** Leading a spiritual life is not impossible. It begins with leading a human life with awareness and love. Today make a vow to enjoy and express your humanness as the surface of your Divinity.

## FEBRUARY 29

*Balance is not a static state but is like a pendulum that swings from side to side.*

**LIVING YOUR YOGA:** We all crave balance. But too often we think balance means perfection. Instead, be grateful for your mistakes and regrets: they give balance to your victories and celebrations.

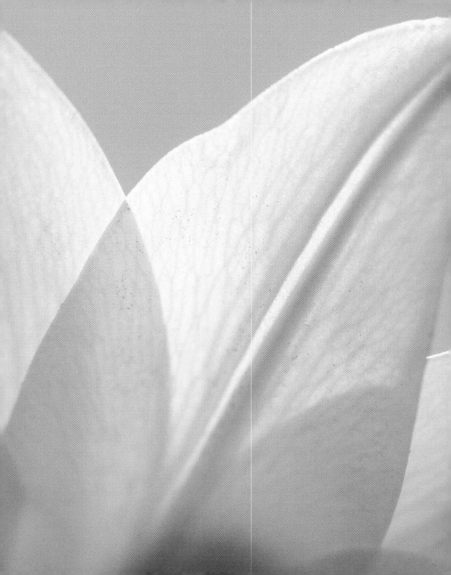

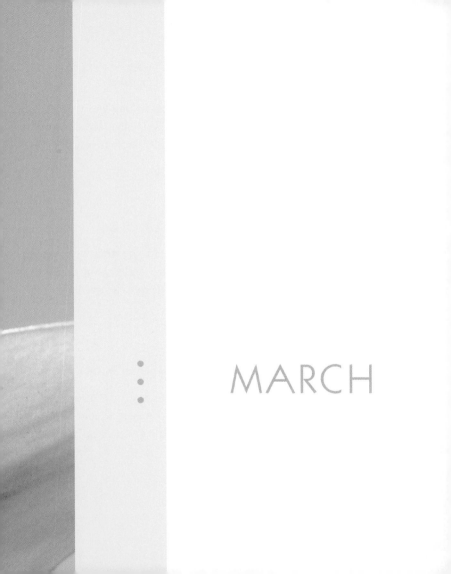

MARCH

## MARCH 1

*Integrity is what you do when no one is looking.*

LIVING YOUR YOGA: To practice yoga, telling the truth is not enough. We need to practice not lying. Today live with integrity by not lying to yourself about one important thing in your life.


## MARCH 2

*Being ourselves is what others really want from us.*

LIVING YOUR YOGA: We often try so hard to be what we think others want us to be. Ironically, what they really want us to do is reveal ourselves. Today have the courage to be yourself.


## MARCH 3

*To understand union, you must understand separation.*

LIVING YOUR YOGA: Union with another can only occur when we fully occupy our place in the world. Let yourself expand to fill your place, so that the coming together with loved ones can be that much sweeter.

## MARCH 4

*The three most important things in life are love, courage, and enthusiasm.*

LIVING YOUR YOGA: Loving yourself and others, taking courage from that, and living each day with enthusiasm are the basis for a happy life. I will step onto my yoga mat today with the intention to love myself and my practice, and to try something difficult with courage and gusto.

## MARCH 5

*There is always a part of us that knows what we need.*

LIVING YOUR YOGA: A sure way to suffer is to deny the knowledge that bubbles up in us from deep inside. Try this: unroll your yoga mat, lie down, and wait for your body to tell you what to do instead of you telling your body what to do. Even if you spend your whole practice time lying there, you are deeply honoring yourself, living in the present, and, at the very least, you will be more rested!

## MARCH 6

*Perfectionism comes from the intellect, not from the heart.*

**LIVING YOUR YOGA:** It is the mind that tells us our asana are not perfect enough, our house is not clean enough, our work is not good enough. The heart knows that perfection is nonexistent. Today do something creative: make up a new asana, write a song, make bread for the first time. Rejoice.

## MARCH 7

*If you are a rose, don't try to be a daisy.*

**LIVING YOUR YOGA:** So you're not tall, with long legs and a flat stomach. You are a rose, and the world needs roses, not just daisies. Today refuse to judge yourself for what you are not. Instead, stand in your own light.

## MARCH 8

*Don't respond to yesterday's bell.*

**LIVING YOUR YOGA:** When we hang out in the past, we miss experiencing the fresh breeze of *this* morning. Regardless of yesterday, notice what arises in your practice today. Enjoy your experiences.

## MARCH 9

*Ego is a shadow cast by the mind.*

LIVING YOUR YOGA: Our favorite mantra is usually "me, me, me."
Find a container you use for drinking water and write the word
*compassion* on it. Then, every time you drink from it today, you
will be reminded to think of opening your heart: toward your own
suffering, toward the suffering of others.

## MARCH 10

*Difficulty is 100 percent subjective.*

LIVING YOUR YOGA: No matter how hard an asana is, there is
someone who finds it easy, and vice versa. Begin today to practice
a pose you find difficult, and keep at it for the next twenty-one
days. Imagine that the pose is easy and you love it.

## MARCH 11

*Come back to the sensations of the breath.*

LIVING YOUR YOGA: Before you answer the phone or take the first
bite of a meal, return for a few seconds to the sensations that
breathing engenders. This will bring you into the present and slow
you down, two things I recommend for a happy life.

## MARCH 12

*Go to your belly.*

**LIVING YOUR YOGA:** When facing a decision today, be it small or large, pause first to pay attention to what you feel in your belly. This "second brain" will never lead you astray.

## MARCH 13

*Hold the difficult as sacred.*

**LIVING YOUR YOGA:** We often take up asana practice to avoid life's difficulties. But it is in the difficulties that we grow. You don't need to like the difficulties that life sends you, but remember that they too are part of the sacred path of evolution. Before you step on your mat today say this aloud: *I hold as sacred the difficulties I may encounter today.*

## MARCH 14

*Postures are questions, not answers.*

**LIVING YOUR YOGA:** Practicing asana is not about getting the right answers but rather about continuing to ask questions: *How am I breathing? Where does my mind wander? How can I create ease in my body right now?* Ask yourself these questions when you practice today.

## MARCH 15

*Yoga is a strategy for a happy life.*

**LIVING YOUR YOGA:** All the main practices of yoga—asana, pranayama, and meditation—are about letting go of suffering, letting go of creating suffering in others, and thereby living a happy life. Today make the decision to let go of something that has been bothering you.

## MARCH 16

*In the state of yoga, there are no distractions.*

LIVING YOUR YOGA: In the swirl of life's events, it is easy to be distracted from what is really important. Today when someone speaks to you, put down what you are doing, turn toward her, and give her your full attention. It will reduce your stress and create connection with her.

## MARCH 17

*Yoga is the conscious choice of the difficult.*

LIVING YOUR YOGA: Get on your yoga mat and choose a pose that is difficult, if not impossible, for you to practice. Practice it anyway. No whining.

## MARCH 18

*Can I be safe and challenged at the same time?*

LIVING YOUR YOGA: Think of something you have been putting off because you are a little afraid of doing it: making a specific phone call, writing a letter, or telling someone your truth. Do it today with an open heart.

## MARCH 19

*What is true for me right now?*

**LIVING YOUR YOGA:** Three times today, stop and ask yourself, *What is true and alive for me right now?* Then live from that understanding.

## MARCH 20

*Honor your divinity; honor the divinity of the other as well.*

**LIVING YOUR YOGA:** At the end of yoga class, we often say *Namaste* to each other. Today say a silent *Namaste* to everyone you see or talk to.

## MARCH 21

*It is not only our actions that matter but also the attitudes behind them.*

**LIVING YOUR YOGA:** Refuse to act today unless you know the clear intention behind your actions.

## March 22
*Yoga practice exposes the deepest parts of ourselves.*

**Living Your Yoga:** Like an onion, we have many layers. During your practice today, use each exhalation to explore another layer of the pose.

## March 23
*Healthy things are sometimes painful, but not all painful things are healthy.*

**Living Your Yoga:** Pay attention to any discomfort you feel today. Is this the pain of health or injury? Is this relationship healthy or just familiar?

## March 24
*Wisdom is knowing which pain is to be endured and which is not.*

**Living Your Yoga:** Beginning students are the most difficult to teach, not because they don't know the poses but because they often cannot discriminate between the pain of opening and the pain of injury. Pay attention to this distinction in your asana practice today.

## MARCH 25

*If I avoid practicing, then everyday things do not have the meaning I want them to have. If I avoid the everyday things, then practice does not have the sweetness it could have.*

**LIVING YOUR YOGA:** No matter how demanding your commitments are, find a few minutes to stretch, breathe, and sit quietly today. No excuses.

## MARCH 26

*Fun can take me away from my life; enjoyment takes me into my life.*

**LIVING YOUR YOGA:** Fun can be something we use to escape from our lives. Enjoyment is the sweetness of noticing your life right now: the sunset, the taste of cool water, the smell of clean sheets. Find something to enjoy right now.

## MARCH 27

*I want freedom in my life, not freedom from it.*

LIVING YOUR YOGA: Sometimes we use yoga practice to escape from what is. This is not freedom. True freedom is the ability to be radically present to what arises, regardless of what it is. Take a vow right now to be willing to live this way. Renew it throughout the day.

## MARCH 28

*To teach is to honor your clarity and truth.*

LIVING YOUR YOGA: No matter how much you know, it touches others when you speak clearly your own truth. Speak to your child or spouse or coworker today from your own knowing.

## MARCH 29

*What am I choosing right now?*

LIVING YOUR YOGA: We get caught up in the habits of perception and action. When you find yourself eating mindlessly or vegging out in front of the television, ask yourself, *What am I choosing right now? Does it enrich my life and the life of the world?*

## MARCH 30
*Whatever you love has the power to transform you.*

LIVING YOUR YOGA: The only way we change is by love. When we love, our heart opens and we become vulnerable to that which we love. Get on your yoga mat and practice the pose you hate the most. Do it with the intention of embracing the pose with love. Notice the difference in your body.


## MARCH 31
*I respect you enough to ask you to respect me.*

LIVING YOUR YOGA: Offer the gift of respect today, especially to your family. Say "please" and "thank you" to them whenever you can, treating them with the politeness that you sometimes reserve for strangers.

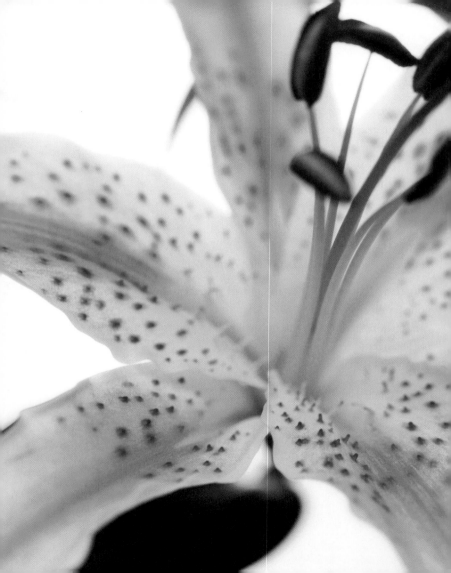

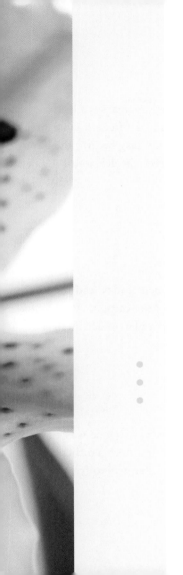

APRIL

## APRIL 1

*There is no such thing as a long life.*

LIVING YOUR YOGA: No matter how many years we live, it will seem to have gone by too quickly. Take a fifteen-minute break today and find something to enjoy: your easy breath, the happy sounds of children playing across the street, the delicious fragrance of a cup of tea.

## APRIL 2

*My main limitation is my own thoughts.*

LIVING YOUR YOGA: Find a quiet moment today and identify a recurring thought that limits your life. Ask yourself, *What would I do if I believed I could?* Then develop a plan to accomplish it.

## APRIL 3

*Choice gives us freedom; freedom allows for choice.*

LIVING YOUR YOGA: Thinking that there is only one way to solve any problem limits the outcome. Today approach a difficult asana with an attitude of freedom; choose another way to try it.

## APRIL 4

*Everything is obvious to God.*

LIVING YOUR YOGA: We all figure things out at our own pace. Today celebrate your evolving understanding of the world and your place in it.

## APRIL 5

*Believing I am right fuels separation and anger.*

LIVING YOUR YOGA: *Righteous anger* is redundant. I can never be angry when I accept that I am wrong. Today when you feel irritated or angry, pause and identify the thought that fuels your belief in your rightness.

## APRIL 6

*You have no control over what others do, only over how you react to it.*

LIVING YOUR YOGA: Control is one of life's greatest illusions. You are not in charge of your children, or partner, or boss. How will you respond to their actions today? You choose: with clarity and empathy, or with anger and disappointment?

## APRIL 7
*My life is right now.*

LIVING YOUR YOGA: Stop looking. Life is already right here.


## APRIL 8
*We only laugh when we sense some truth; lies are never funny.*

LIVING YOUR YOGA: We laugh when we connect to the truth of something. Today when you laugh, spend a moment considering what is true for you.


## APRIL 9
*Information is not sufficient for a well-lived life.*

LIVING YOUR YOGA: Unfortunately, you can know all the facts and still be miserable. Open your heart and feel the moment as well as understand it.


## APRIL 10
*Yoga practice is important, not serious.*

LIVING YOUR YOGA: What if your asana practice was your play? Practice is too important not to be joyous. Play today!

## APRIL 11

*A river requires banks as well as flowing water.*

**LIVING YOUR YOGA:** In each asana you practice today, find which parts of your body are held steady and firm, and which are soft and yielding. Balancing these two elements creates harmony in asana and in life.

## APRIL 12

*We can know everything and still be unhappy.*

**LIVING YOUR YOGA:** Knowledge is important but it is not enough. Remember that your happiness lies deep within you, whether or not things on the surface are falling apart. As you go through your day, stop, take a deep breath, and remember this, especially during the challenging moments.

## APRIL 13

*Today I will spend fifteen minutes doing nothing.*

**LIVING YOUR YOGA:** Find a quiet place. If it is outdoors, lie down and gaze at the sky. If it is indoors, lie down and just listen to the sounds around you. Each moment is full. Stay for fifteen minutes and then continue your day, a little more relaxed.

## APRIL 14

*Nothing can be true if it is also harmful.*

LIVING YOUR YOGA: Remember today that your words leave a residue. Choose them carefully so you can speak the truth with sweetness.

## APRIL 15

*My beliefs are just my beliefs.*

LIVING YOUR YOGA: Beliefs are really only important because we believe them. Ask yourself right now, *Can I honor my beliefs and yet understand they are not a true reflection of reality?*

## APRIL 16

*When I judge another, I limit that person as well as myself.*

LIVING YOUR YOGA: To judge is to put self or other in a box. Focus today on your actions. Ask yourself, *Are my actions kind? Do they support my values?* Just for today, refuse to judge yourself as good or bad.

## APRIL 17

*Shifting and giving in are not the same thing.*

LIVING YOUR YOGA: Today when you feel pressured to make a different choice in some small thing, focus on the other person's point of view. If you can, shift to his point of view. This is not the same as giving in. Shifting your viewpoint requires strength; giving in comes from fear.

## APRIL 18

*We begin again every day.*

LIVING YOUR YOGA: Every day you are a beginning yoga student. Begin again right now.

## APRIL 19

*My practice is not limited by location but by intention.*

LIVING YOUR YOGA: You do not need a mat to practice yoga. Today repeat this intention to yourself whenever you can: *I can practice yoga right here, right now.* This intention will transform your day.

## APRIL 20
*Time is big.*

LIVING YOUR YOGA: Our belief that we don't have enough time is false. We have all the time there is to have. We just fill it up with too much. Today when you feel rushed, say aloud, *Time is big,* and notice yourself relax.

## APRIL 21
*Let go into your strength.*

LIVING YOUR YOGA: We think that strength is about being able to push something away or hold something back. We have great reserves of strength, which can be used in different ways. Inhale, and let go into the strength you already have to do Adho Mukha Vrksasana (Handstand) or to create an hour with no commitments.

## APRIL 22
*Responding appropriately is an art.*

LIVING YOUR YOGA: Do you overdo some things and underdo others? For today, see if you can apply just enough effort to each task. This requires that you stay present.

## APRIL 23

*The greatest strength we possess is the unwillingness to give up hope.*

**LIVING YOUR YOGA:** Strength is not always obvious. Think about a challenge you face in your life. Sit down for five minutes today and imagine that situation from a hopeful viewpoint. Then act as if that hope were an actuality.

## APRIL 24

*Strength and rigidity are not the same thing.*

**LIVING YOUR YOGA:** The ability to bend and flow without losing your center is the manifestation of strength. Practice five Surya Namaskar (Sun Salutations) today with this in mind.

## APRIL 25

*Practicing requires listening to your body.*

**LIVING YOUR YOGA:** Too often we practice by telling our body what to do. Today when you are on your yoga mat, spend more time in each pose listening to your body instead.

## APRIL 26
*How we deal with conflict reflects our understanding of yoga.*

LIVING YOUR YOGA: What do you do in a conflict? Demand your way or melt in fear? Today when you find yourself in a small conflict, stand in Tadasana (Mountain Pose) and open your heart before you speak.

## APRIL 27
*What would my life be like without this recurring thought?*

LIVING YOUR YOGA: We all have thoughts that repeat time and again. Today when one of these thoughts arises, notice it, take a breath, and consciously let it go.

## APRIL 28
*Acceptance and acknowledgement are not the same.*

LIVING YOUR YOGA: Some things are unacceptable, such as child abuse or cruelty to animals. But they exist and therefore we must acknowledge them. Today I will acknowledge the evil in the world and, at the same time, I commit to never accepting it.

## APRIL 29

*Attachment is what arises in us when we don't get
our preference.*

**LIVING YOUR YOGA:** We all have preferences: the blue shirt over the red, tea instead of coffee, yoga over wrestling. Preferences do not limit our life. What limits it is the feeling that arises when we don't get our way. This feeling is attachment, which constricts enjoyment. Today when the feeling of attachment arises, notice it and consciously let it go. What happened?

## APRIL 30

*How we face the inevitability of our death shapes our life
right now.*

**LIVING YOUR YOGA:** Our culture denies death. But denying our mortality actually reduces the sweetness of life in this moment. Today sit down for a few moments, consider that you will die, and feel the sadness that accompanies your understanding. Then stand up and go about your day with enthusiasm and an open heart.

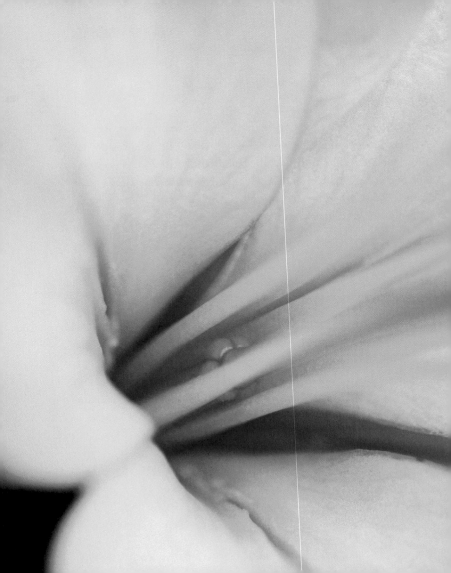

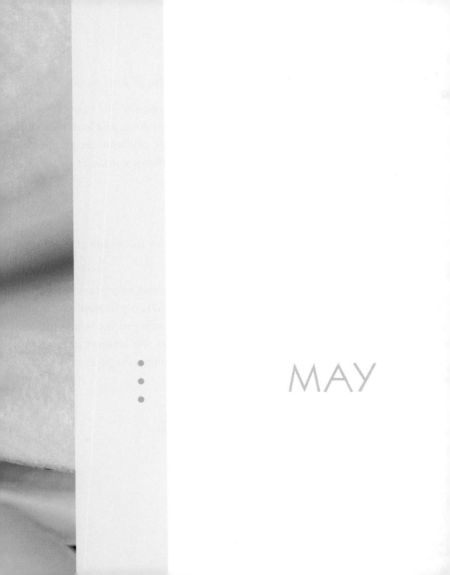

MAY

## MAY 1

*Clarity about money is just another form of yoga practice.*

**LIVING YOUR YOGA:** Our beliefs about money often contribute to our suffering. Plan a time right now to sit down and look with clarity at your financial life. When you do, celebrate the things you like and make a plan to deal with the things you don't.

## MAY 2

*What I bring to my yoga mat is really my whole life at this moment.*

**LIVING YOUR YOGA:** Mood, thoughts, and beliefs are as much a part of yoga practice as your body is. When you step on the mat today, take a deep breath and pay attention to the whole of your being practicing. When you do this, you will be more present and less at the mercy of your ever-changing moods, thoughts, and beliefs.

## MAY 3

*Being aware can become a habit.*

LIVING YOUR YOGA: Right now, take a deep breath and settle into this very moment. Look around. However familiar the surroundings, find something new to look at, or see a familiar thing in a new way. Cultivate this practice through the day whenever possible.

## MAY 4

*To change the body affects the mind.*

LIVING YOUR YOGA: When we change the body, we affect the mind, whether by asana, breathing, or meditation. Before you practice, spend some quiet moments noticing the state of your mind; at the end of your practice do the same.

## MAY 5

*My breath exists only in the present, never in the past*
*or in the future.*

LIVING YOUR YOGA: Sit quietly with your back tall and chest open. Close your eyes and breathe ten long, slow breaths. Note afterward how your mind has settled a bit. Then say to yourself, *When I pay attention to my breath, I am always in the present.*

## MAY 6

*There is nowhere to go where God is not.*

LIVING YOUR YOGA: An old story explains the plight of a drunkard who seeks refuge in a temple to drink. When castigated by the priest for defiling the sanctity of the temple, he says, "I'm so sorry; if you will just tell me where God isn't, I will go and drink there." Today open your heart to the Divine in all beings, in all places, and in all things.


## MAY 7

*The mind is a mixed blessing.*

LIVING YOUR YOGA: Although the mind can be creative and insightful, it sees a small slice of reality, which it attempts to impose on others. For today, note how easily your "trusted" mind is disturbed, distracted, or angry. Then breathe and remember that you are not your thoughts but much, much more.

## MAY 8
*Beliefs are rigid thoughts.*

LIVING YOUR YOGA: Beliefs are thoughts that get repeated enough to take on a kind of internal structure. No belief is the truth; it is only a belief. As a practice, allow yourself to let go of one tiny belief today.

## MAY 9
*Yoga is a practice of observation and faith.*

LIVING YOUR YOGA: When we observe as clearly as possible and have faith in the efficacy of our practice, we are living yoga. Take this awareness onto your mat today.

## MAY 10
*Pay attention.*

LIVING YOUR YOGA: Today's practice is to do one thing at a time: turn off the car radio and drive; talk on the phone without working on the computer; eat without watching television. Notice that when you pay attention, you can enjoy what you are doing—life— much more.

## MAY 11
*Nothing is missing.*

LIVING YOUR YOGA: Sometimes we think, *If I only I had _____, then I would be complete*. But there is nothing missing in your soul. Today repeat this Mantra for Daily Living quietly to yourself whenever you remember: *Nothing is missing.*

## MAY 12
*Am I here?*

LIVING YOUR YOGA: How often are we really where we are? Don't we eat lunch and discuss dinner, or plan Thanksgiving and worry about Christmas? Make a pledge today to focus on what you are doing or thinking with your whole being. Each time you forget, come back to right now.

## MAY 13
*Relax and renew.*

LIVING YOUR YOGA: Find twenty minutes to lie down and put your feet up. Close your eyes and allow your fatigue to surface and fly away. Then savor this state of sweet ease fully before you roll to the side and carefully get up.

## MAY 14

*When you open to life, you are helping people you will never meet.*

LIVING YOUR YOGA: You make decisions every day, and they have an effect on the world. When you are present and make choices from this state of mind, the effect of what you choose creates ever-widening ripples that will help beings you may never meet. Be present as you make decisions today.

## MAY 15

*Heart up, brain down.*

LIVING YOUR YOGA: When all else fails you today, sit or stand with awareness, and slightly lower your chin to bring your brain down and lift your chest to bring your heart up. This will help create in you a state of yoga. Now you will be more likely to choose skillful words and actions.

## MAY 16

*Control is a dangerous illusion.*

**LIVING YOUR YOGA:** I have found that my need to control things is based on fear and is a strategy for feeling safe in the world. Today examine one small aspect of your life that you feel you need to control. Consider your need and what lies beneath it. Then make a decision to let go of controlling it. Breathe as you do.

## MAY 17

*If you are confused, be the best confused person on Earth.*

**LIVING YOUR YOGA:** When we are confused, we feel agitated. This agitation has more to do with what we *tell* ourselves about being confused rather than actually being confused. Today when you feel confused, stop, take a breath and let yourself feel totally confused. You will smile. Being confused is not the problem; our reaction to being confused is the problem.

## MAY 18

*Am I doing the right things for the wrong reasons?*

**LIVING YOUR YOGA:** To live an authentic life, we must live from our own integrity. No matter how laudable your choice today, if it is made for someone else's reasons, then it will not make your life more wonderful. Choose from your heart today with courage and love.

## MAY 19

*Whatever we experienced as a child, we consider normal.*

**LIVING YOUR YOGA:** What we learned about love and relationships from our childhood feels normal. But just because something feels familiar doesn't mean it is healthy. Spend five minutes today quietly reflecting on one of your relationships. Does it enrich your life? If you find that it doesn't, consider what changes you need to make so the relationship feeds you.

## MAY 20

*Open and receive.*

**LIVING YOUR YOGA:** Today when someone offers you something—an inviting smile, a warm cup of tea, or a chance to go ahead in a line, receive it completely and without reservation.

## May 21

*Patience doesn't exist.*

LIVING YOUR YOGA: We are either in the flow with the speed of what is happening or we are impatient. Being patient is an attempt to cover our own impatience. For today, try moving at life's pace. If it is moving too fast for your comfort, consider reducing what you have planned for the day by 10 percent.

## May 22

*Asana teaches us how to push away and let go at the same time.*

LIVING YOUR YOGA: Step onto your mat and practice Utthita Trikonasana (Extended Triangle Pose). Notice how your feet and legs push the floor away, while your hips and back let go as you extend to the side. The legs say no, and the hips and back say yes. Knowing when to say yes and when to say no make life more satisfying.

## MAY 23
*Nothing attracts the tongue more than a rough tooth.*

LIVING YOUR YOGA: What is difficult draws our attention. While practicing your favorite asana today, notice that your mind goes to the most difficult part of the pose. Instead, just for fun, focus on what is easiest about the pose and breathe gently. When you come out, notice how pleasant you feel.


## MAY 24
*L.G.O. (Life goes on.)*

LIVING YOUR YOGA: This is the first Mantra for Daily Living that I taught my three children. I wanted it to remind us that most of our agitations and disappointments disappear quickly. Keep your perspective today when you misplace something, or forget the milk at the store, or find a pose difficult that used to be easy. Say aloud, *L.G.O.,* and smile.

## MAY 25

*Make your inner growth your top priority and everything else will follow.*

**LIVING YOUR YOGA:** No one has any "extra" time. Even so, set aside time today: meditate for five minutes, practice three asana, and lie in Savasana (Basic Relaxation Pose) for twenty minutes. With this foundation, you will change the world.

## MAY 26

*There is nothing to do; just* being *is enough.*

**LIVING YOUR YOGA:** Find a quiet place and lie in Savasana (Basic Relaxation Pose). Support your head, neck, and knees. Cover yourself with a light blanket, and close your eyes. Rest for at least fifteen minutes. Know that you being there is enough for the Universe right now; you don't need to do something, help anyone, or produce anything. You are enough.

## MAY 27

*Life itself holds all the answers.*

LIVING YOUR YOGA: One of the most effective ways to learn to live well is to observe life itself. At the end of your day today, just before sleep, ask yourself, *What did I learn about my life today?* Whatever the answer, rejoice in your awareness.

## MAY 28

*Your child belongs to herself.*

LIVING YOUR YOGA: As much as we want to make life perfect for our child, her life is hers, and helping her and you understand this is the most important job you can do as a parent. Remember today to live the awareness that your life belongs to you and your child's to her.

## MAY 29

*I actually own nothing, therefore I am the steward of everything.*

LIVING YOUR YOGA: What would the world be like if we treated everything as something we had borrowed, something we had to give back? Since we do, indeed, have to give back everything when we die, today treat yourself, everyone you meet, nature, animals, and all objects that you handle with the respect due them as things borrowed.

## MAY 30

*Make friends with your fears because they shape your life.*

LIVING YOUR YOGA: We put things into two categories: what we love and what we fear. Today spend a quiet moment to clarify a fear that frequently arises in your mind. Give this fear an inward *Namaste,* not because you like it, but to honor the power that this fear has to shape your life. Allow the fear to relax if only a little bit.

## MAY 31

*I can only be afraid if I am thinking about the future.*

**LIVING YOUR YOGA:** Even in moments of greatest danger, we are not afraid if we focus on exactly what we must do in that moment. Fear arises when we think about what might happen or what could have happened. Today when you feel afraid, note that you are thinking of the future. Take a breath (or several), and settle into now.

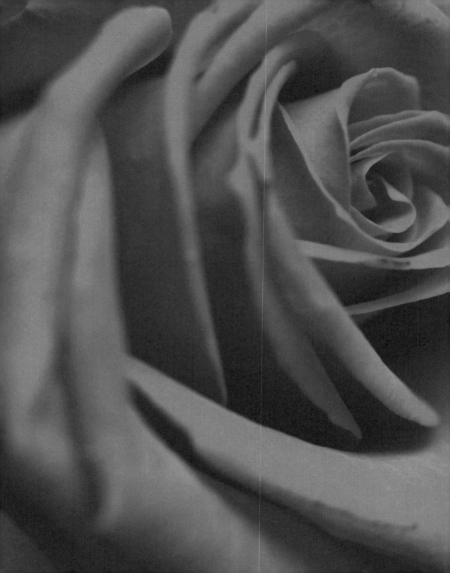

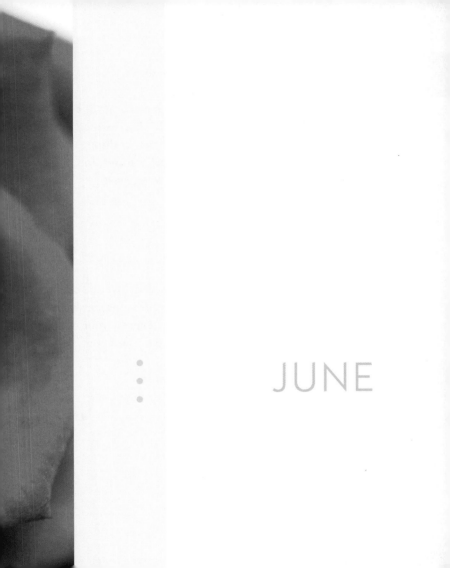

JUNE

## JUNE 1

*There is no such thing as wasted love.*

**LIVING YOUR YOGA:** When a relationship ends, one or both parties may feel that their love was "wasted." But love can never be wasted; it is embedded in our being and fuels us through our whole life. Right now, spend a moment and feel gratitude for all the love you have given and all the love you have received.

## JUNE 2

*To live with courage is the highest form of practice.*

**LIVING YOUR YOGA:** It is interesting that both love and courage are said to reside in the heart. When we live by consciously choosing courage, we express life's spirit. Today express your courage by choosing something difficult to say or do. It need only be a small thing, but it will open your heart.

## JUNE 3
*Security doesn't exist.*

LIVING YOUR YOGA: We all long for security: from loneliness, from fear, from illness. Yet the great irony is that nothing is secure enough to last, even with the best planning. Sit quietly for a few minutes. Inhale slowly, and as you exhale let yourself settle into the awareness that all is fleeting. This awareness is the only security.

## JUNE 4
*True freedom can never be taken away.*

LIVING YOUR YOGA: Even if you are in jail, your inner freedom lives. Today when you hear yourself saying you are "stuck" in some way, remember that true freedom can never be touched.

## JUNE 5
*Growing old is not a mistake.*

LIVING YOUR YOGA: We live in a youth-oriented culture. We are given the message that growing older is to be avoided. Today celebrate your age, whatever it is. (If it's your birthday, Happy Birthday!)

## JUNE 6

*Am I lovable? How I answer this question will affect me every day.*

LIVING YOUR YOGA: Today when you lie in Savasana (Basic Relaxation Pose), remind yourself that you are the product of the love of the Universe. See this in yourself and see in it others throughout the day.

## JUNE 7

*Our commitment is to the process, not the goal.*

LIVING YOUR YOGA: Commitment to a goal can make us rigid. Instead, recommit today to the *process* of getting to your goal. This commitment to process will allow new information to shape your learning on the way to your goal.

## JUNE 8

*Letting go is the hardest asana.*

**LIVING YOUR YOGA:** Life is about letting go: of every exhalation, of the day as we fall asleep, of our children as they grow up and leave home. When we resist letting go, we are resisting the flow of life itself. What can you let go of right now?

## JUNE 9

*Breath is the doorway in.*

**LIVING YOUR YOGA:** Lie comfortably on your yoga mat in Savasana (Basic Relaxation Pose), with your head, neck, shoulders, and knees lightly supported. Bring your attention to your breath, specifically your inhalation. With each one, allow your awareness to be taken in deeper and deeper. After ten to fifteen breaths, release your breath to its own intelligence, its own rhythm, but stay with this deeper awareness.

## JUNE 10

*Being present is not difficult, remembering to be present is.*

LIVING YOUR YOGA: When you finish reading these words, stop where you are and be aware of what is happening in your body, of the sensations of breath, of the noises around you, of the feelings that arise within you. Can you bring this quality of awareness to all that you do? It is not a hard process but one that is overcome by busy mind again and again. Remember to practice this exercise whenever you can.

## JUNE 11

*Separation and union happen at the same time.*

LIVING YOUR YOGA: Stand on your yoga mat and practice Utthita Trikonasana (Extended Triangle Pose). Keep your breath flowing as you move into the pose, and focus on each limb of your body. Notice how your arms move away from each other and how one leg rotates away from the other. Inhale and come up. Now practice the pose and focus on your body as a whole. Notice how both experiences are true for you, on the yoga mat and off.

## JUNE 12

*With perspective comes wisdom.*

**LIVING YOUR YOGA:** Recall an event from your youth when you felt that the outcome was "life or death," such as making the team or having a date to the prom. With your current perspective, note how your interpretation has changed. Now think of a current conflict and know that in the future you will have a different perspective about it as well. Understanding that everything is subject to change is wisdom.

## JUNE 13

*The ability to laugh at yourself is a sign of mental health.*

**LIVING YOUR YOGA:** Today open to the experience of laughing at something you say or do and relish your ability to do so.

## JUNE 14

*Only the soft earth absorbs the rain.*

**LIVING YOUR YOGA:** The practice of yoga is not about becoming more flexible but rather about becoming softer so you can fully receive life. Make time for Savasana (Basic Relaxation Pose) today. Support your head, neck, and knees, and cover your eyes. Receive the moment through your senses: sensations, sounds, and thoughts. Soften to your life as you experience it in this moment. Stay at least fifteen minutes before rolling over and getting up.

## JUNE 15

*I cannot understand the Universe with my brain; I can only experience it with my heart.*

**LIVING YOUR YOGA:** We are surrounded by mysteries. Where is the Universe? What is the Universe? Why is the Universe? Even the wisest people cannot answer these questions definitely. But you can decide to open your heart to the Universe today and welcome it, even though your understanding is incomplete.

## JUNE 16

*Reality is just one point of view.*

**LIVING YOUR YOGA:** Reality is fascinating, confusing, and difficult all at once. Today become a "reality sociologist," and observe yourself and those around you. What will happen next? Be curious, and notice how you take things a little more lightly.


## JUNE 17

*Only you can give yourself permission to be happy.*

**LIVING YOUR YOGA:** We grow up when we realize that no one is going to tap us on the shoulder and say, *Now you have done enough so you can be happy.* Take a deep breath and make the decision that you will connect with your own happiness for the next five minutes. At the end of this time, make the commitment for the next five minutes, and then the next. Know that your ability to be happy lies within you, only you, and is not dependent on your circumstances.

## JUNE 18

*Don't trust anyone who doesn't like garlic.*

**LIVING YOUR YOGA:** Living life to the fullest means that we embrace the strong sensations as well as the gentle ones. Today allow yourself to taste a food you usually don't, or think a thought you are afraid to entertain, or smile at someone you don't like. Embrace the spiciness of life.

## JUNE 19

*Listening is the greatest gift we can give others.*

**LIVING YOUR YOGA:** Listening is being willing to be changed by what we hear. Today listen to everyone without planning what to say or thinking about something else while they are talking. Not only will this help you stay present, but it also will transform your relationships.

## JUNE 20

*If you are not comfortable in your body, you will not be comfortable anywhere.*

**LIVING YOUR YOGA:** Sometimes we blame our unhappiness on where we are instead of what is going on inside us. When you practice yoga today, find a pose in which you are happy in your body just as you are. Then remember that feeling throughout the day.

## JUNE 21

*Conflict arises from a lack of commitment.*

**LIVING YOUR YOGA:** Too often we make a decision and then find we can't stick to it. We waffle; we argue with ourselves; we feel irritated. Today examine a decision that you feel unable to keep, contemplating if you are truly committed to that decision. What is holding you back from that commitment?

## JUNE 22

*The mind is not a thing; what you think will change.*

**LIVING YOUR YOGA:** The mind reflects how everything changes. Think back to how your opinion on any number of things has changed. Practice this Mantra for Daily Living today: *Everything changes.* This will give you some freedom from the tyranny of your thoughts.

## JUNE 23

*The foundation of the house of yoga is compassion.*

**LIVING YOUR YOGA:** No matter what advanced asana you can do, if you don't practice it with compassion, then it is not as transformative as it could be. Try this: Sit quietly, and breathe slowly and deeply for five minutes. As you do, become aware of spaciousness within you. With each inhalation, breathe compassion for yourself and all of your life choices into this space. As you exhale, breathe compassion into a weary world. Stay with this practice for ten more minutes. Remember it as you go about your day.

## JUNE 24

*The attitude that you bring to the mat will shape your poses.*

**LIVING YOUR YOGA:** We give too much power to the poses to change us and too little power to ourselves to change the poses. Today before you practice asana, do something you really love: bake cookies, or sing a song, or play with your child. Notice how it affects your joy. Then take this joy to the mat, and watch what happens to your practice.

## JUNE 25

*There is no escape.*

**LIVING YOUR YOGA:** Longing for escape is a waste of time. Even if we go on an exotic vacation, we still bring our thoughts with us. The only true escape is through transformation, and the only true transformation is freedom from thoughts. Today when you remember to, say to yourself this Mantra for Daily Living: *I have thoughts but I am not my thoughts.*

## JUNE 26

*No one is coming.*

**LIVING YOUR YOGA:** Salvation does not come from someone else; it comes from opening your heart to self, to others, and to Divinity. Lie on your back over a pillow, with your knees bent and arms out to the sides, so that your chest is comfortably supported to open. Breathe ten gentle breaths with an open heart.

## JUNE 27
*Other people are not the problem.*

**LIVING YOUR YOGA:** As long as I believe that others are the source of my suffering, I will continue to suffer. Others may be the stimulus for my suffering, but they are never the cause. My thoughts are the cause. Today remember that others are not the problem whenever you can, and it will soften your day.

## JUNE 28
*If I am focusing on learning, then I never make a mistake; I just learn a lot.*

**LIVING YOUR YOGA:** I once owned a yoga studio that I sold after four months. Others asked me if I felt like a failure because I sold it so quickly. I told them that, on the contrary, I felt like a success because I learned that I didn't want to own a yoga studio. Today reframe what you call a failure as a learning experience. Then notice how different you feel.

## JUNE 29

*I have learned to love some people in spite of themselves.*

**LIVING YOUR YOGA:** Not everyone acts as we would wish. This obvious fact can interfere with our ability to love them. Today observe those you love and see their faults as what makes them the very person you love. Say this Mantra for Daily Living to yourself, *I love you in spite of yourself; I love myself in spite of myself,* and smile.

## JUNE 30

*Chocolate is one of the sacraments.*

**LIVING YOUR YOGA:** Being truly alive to our sensations is to be truly alive to life. Sit in a quiet place and take a bite of your favorite chocolate. Hold it on your tongue; let it melt slightly. Taste it fully. Enjoy the smell. It is not the chocolate that is the practice; it is the ability to be fully alive to each moment. Cultivate this practice today.

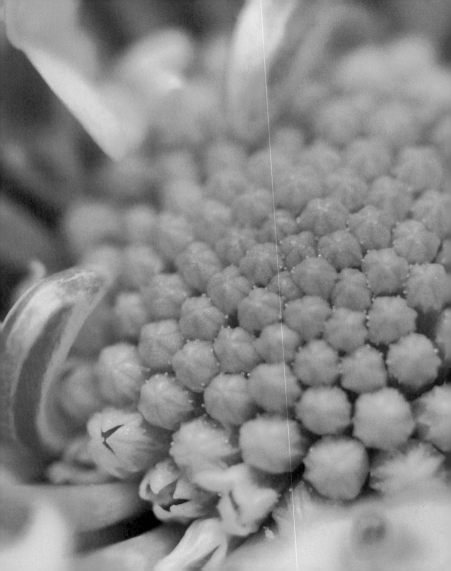

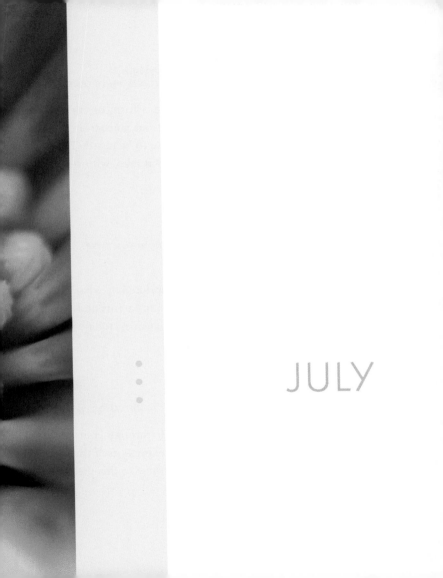

JULY

## JULY 1

*Fighting to overcome your resistance creates more resistance.*

**LIVING YOUR YOGA:** Resistance is just a form of energy. When resistance arises today, hold it as a precious voice from your inner wisdom. Sit quietly and allow that voice to be heard. Then decide with clarity what action, if any, you will take, with resistance as your companion.

## JULY 2

*You are raising your grandchildren by how you raise your children.*

**LIVING YOUR YOGA:** Each of us was imprinted by what I call emotional DNA, which we received from our parents and family. We act directly from that imprinting. Consider today what your actions are teaching those around you.

## JULY 3

*Your body is the vehicle for your spirit's expression in the world.*

**LIVING YOUR YOGA:** You experience life through your body. And without a doubt, your spirit can only express itself through your body. Today say a silent prayer of gratitude to this precious body that expresses your spirit.

## JULY 4

*If you have a yoga mat, you are more likely to practice.*

LIVING YOUR YOGA: Practicing on your own is supported by your commitment to it. Right now: roll out your yoga mat and practice three poses.

## JULY 5

*We can become too used to what is usual and miss what is important.*

LIVING YOUR YOGA: Today on your yoga mat, choose to practice a strong twisting pose. As you do, visualize that the pose is untwisting the knots that bind you, so you can experience with freshness that which is truly important.

## JULY 6

*Give the world the gift of a relaxed, loving, and present person—you!*

LIVING YOUR YOGA: End your asana practice today with a twenty-minute Savasana (Basic Relaxation Pose), followed by a few minutes in reflection. The effects will change you and contribute to the peace of the world.

## July 7

*Instead of getting something from my yoga practice today, what can I give to my practice?*

**LIVING YOUR YOGA:** Step on your mat today and ask yourself, *What can I give to my practice right now? My attention? My faith? My concentration?*

## July 8

*Finding God and finding Self are the same thing.*

**LIVING YOUR YOGA:** Ultimately, yoga practice is about recognizing the union of Self and Divinity. Sit quietly this morning. As you inhale, invite Divinity within. With each exhalation, share your Self with the world. Practice this for ten minutes, and live it the rest of your day.

## July 9

*Inhale, exhale.*

**LIVING YOUR YOGA:** You will experience at least one stressful moment today. When you do, remember to inhale and to exhale. Breathing will slow you down, so you will be more likely to make the choices you enjoy in your life.

## JULY 10

*Standing on your own two feet is the most important asana.*

**LIVING YOUR YOGA:** Step on your yoga mat and stand in Tadasana (Mountain Pose). Make your feet parallel, ask your thighs to roll inward, slightly lift your breastbone, while slightly dropping your chin. Like a mountain, root your feet into the earth, but let your heart soar to the heavens. Breathe five slow breaths. Now take this openhearted rootedness into your life.

## JULY 11

*Jump.*

**LIVING YOUR YOGA:** Pick something you have been waffling about and *jump!* In other words, go ahead, take a chance, try something new or something you're unsure about. Notice how liberated you feel.

## JULY 12

*Whenever we give our full attention, we are practicing.*

**LIVING YOUR YOGA:** Yoga is not a small practice. It can become as big as you wish. Today bring your full attention to whatever it is that you are doing, and you will be living your yoga.

## JULY 13

*My words reflect my thoughts; my thoughts reflect my beliefs; and my beliefs run my life.*

LIVING YOUR YOGA: Today pay attention to your words, especially those such as *should, have to,* and *you made me.* These words reflect your unexamined thoughts. They spring from your beliefs about the world. Just for today, do not speak or think these words, and see what happens.

## JULY 14

*Planning ahead is both absolutely necessary and completely impossible.*

LIVING YOUR YOGA: Before you start your day, spend ten minutes making a specific plan for how you will spend each hour of your day. At the end of the day, notice how you followed the plan and how you did not. Remember, planning enables us to focus, but forcing the plan creates rigidity. Celebrate your ability to plan for flexibility.

## JULY 15

*Whatever I spend my time doing is what I am committed to in my life.*

**LIVING YOUR YOGA:** Notice what you spend your time doing. That is what you are truly committed to. Are you happy with this commitment? Ask yourself, *What needs change and what merits celebration about how I spend my time each day?*

## JULY 16

*Every breath is an experiment.*

**LIVING YOUR YOGA:** Even things that we take for granted are unique. When you practice your asana today, stay present with each breath. Note how each one is different and has something to teach.

## JULY 17

*It is a miracle that every day all my cells agree to be me for one more day.*

**LIVING YOUR YOGA:** Today when you lie down to practice Savasana (Basic Relaxation Pose), begin by thanking your whole body for supporting your consciousness.

## JULY 18

*How can I stand on my head when the Earth is spinning though space at 60,000 miles an hour?*

**LIVING YOUR YOGA:** Our existence in the world is such a mystery. Choose this Mantra of Daily Living to repeat to yourself: *Today I will practice with love and courage, even though I don't understand how my life will turn out.*

## JULY 19

*Simple and easy are not the same thing.*

**LIVING YOUR YOGA:** Adho Mukha Svanasana (Downward-Facing Dog Pose) is a simple action, but it is not easy to perform with love and consistency. Honor yourself today for the so-called simple things you have chosen in your life. Remember, they are usually not so easy.

## JULY 20

*Worrying is a way to avoid what is so by thinking about what could be.*

**LIVING YOUR YOGA:** We all worry. When we do, we are not really living in the present. Today, when you find yourself worrying, say this Mantra for Daily Living: *I notice that I am worrying now; I choose instead to be present.*

## JULY 21

*I am not the general contractor for the Universe.*

**LIVING YOUR YOGA:** It is easy to try to take over responsibility for more than is ours. Today make a commitment to remember that the choices your loved ones make are theirs.

## JULY 22

*I am always right; you are always right. Now what?*

**LIVING YOUR YOGA:** If you focus on who is right in a conflict, you waste everyone's time. If you have a conflict today, focus instead on how to get everyone's needs met in a spirit of mutuality. Open your heart and be creative.

## JULY 23

*The fundamental truth of the Universe is that everything, from electrons to planets, exists in relationship to everything else. What is the quality of my relationships?*

**LIVING YOUR YOGA:** Even if you are marooned on a desert island, you are still in relationship with yourself. Ask yourself, *What is my intention with my relationships today? Connection with others? Or power over them?* For today, take a breath before you speak to your loved ones. As you talk with them, hold an intention for mutuality.

## JULY 24

*We all need the same things: safety, love, respect, and laughter.*

**LIVING YOUR YOGA:** How can you contribute to your own safety, love, respect, and laughter today? How can you help to meet those needs in others?

## JULY 25

*Respecting life in all its forms is the fundamental sacred act.*

**LIVING YOUR YOGA:** There is no life that is not holy. Respect the life force in bugs that cross your path, flowers that brighten your bedroom, and each person that you see around you.

## JULY 26

*Judging me, positively or negatively, puts me in a box.*

**LIVING YOUR YOGA:** Labeling me as *bad* or *beautiful* is a judgment that makes it harder for me to change in your eyes. Today practice your yoga by telling others what they did or said that enriched your life instead of how you have defined them.

## JULY 27

*My body craves consistency; my mind craves change.*

**LIVING YOUR YOGA:** To balance these cravings, bring newness to your body and consistency to your mind. Today, in Utthita Triko-nasana (Extended Triangle Pose), find a new sensation in your body, while your mind is as steady and reflective as when you are in Savasana (Basic Relaxation Pose). This is the practice of yoga.

## JULY 28

*A juicy red apple is the Universe showing us elegance and simplicity.*

**LIVING YOUR YOGA:** Pick up an apple, feel its firmness, notice its shape, smell its fragrance. If you wish, bite into its sweet white flesh. What a celebration!

## JULY 29

*Few things are as satisfying as fresh, clean sheets and someone to share them with.*

**LIVING YOUR YOGA:** Make your bed with line-dried sheets that you iron. When you crawl in, revel in the sensation and comfort they give you. Consciously receive the bounty of the moment. This is a practice.

## JULY 30

*What my senses tell me is only part of the truth.*

**LIVING YOUR YOGA:** Scientists tell us that we perceive very little of the reality around us. Today cultivate the understanding that you do not have the whole picture about everything. Breathe in humility, breathe out compassion.

## JULY 31

*Pick three poses you love and do them every day.*

**LIVING YOUR YOGA:** Practice does not have to be arduous and unpleasant. Begin today's practice with three poses that you love. See where this takes you.

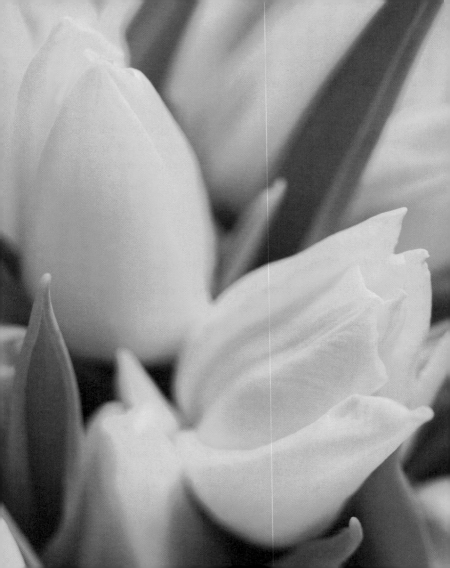

AUGUST

## AUGUST 1

*No one knows my mind, not even me.*

**LIVING YOUR YOGA:** Scientists say that most of our mind is unconscious. For today, know that your thoughts do not totally reflect what is alive in you. Be willing to lovingly distrust your thoughts.

## AUGUST 2

*Fun is when you pay them; work is when they pay you.*

**LIVING YOUR YOGA:** Sometimes we take yoga too seriously, and it stops being fun. Today when you take a yoga class, remember that you chose it: you are willing to pay for it with time and money. Enjoy!

## AUGUST 3

*The simplest vacation is a walk with a friend.*

**LIVING YOUR YOGA:** Plan a walk today with a friend. Enjoy the conversation, the rhythmic movement of your steps, and the fresh air. Note how your mood has lifted when you return.

## AUGUST 4

*May I live as if everything matters, knowing it doesn't.*

**LIVING YOUR YOGA:** If you don't care about anything because it's all impermanent, your life will be dry. If you care too much, your life will lack the wisdom of perspective. Today observe yourself, and remember to balance both detachment and interest in your life.

## AUGUST 5

*It is not possible to do everything or have everything. It is possible to be everything.*

**LIVING YOUR YOGA:** Are you running around trying to accomplish everything or acquire everything? I suggest that you sit quietly for ten minutes and be totally all that you are.

## AUGUST 6

*Nothing remains the same.*

**LIVING YOUR YOGA:** At some time during the day, stop whatever you are doing and look out the window. It is not the same scene as yesterday. Find one new thing to notice or hear, then return to your task with freshness.

## AUGUST 7

*The only people who seem to be done with everything are dead, and we don't even know about them.*

LIVING YOUR YOGA: Today notice your tendency to want to finish everything and make everything perfect. To experience working with more ease, pick a task and commit to doing it for ten minutes. Then leave it and come back to it during the coming days, but still only for ten minutes at a time. Revel in both how the task gets done and how you don't need to be done all at once.

## AUGUST 8

*Trust means I have faith in my ability to survive and thrive.*

LIVING YOUR YOGA: We want to trust others, but we are afraid they will let us down. Today instead of focusing on trusting others, remember that there is something bigger: trust your ability to be okay even if things are not okay.

## AUGUST 9

*I want to live my life so that when I'm dying I will say, Thank God, it's time to go.*

LIVING YOUR YOGA: Even if you live to be 100, life will still probably feel short. Live today fully, with all its pains and joys. Enjoy your life right now.

## AUGUST 10

*Every chance you have, dance to music you love.*

LIVING YOUR YOGA: Sometimes we put off enjoyment until we have finished the term paper, the project at work, or cleaning the house. Given the uncertainty of life, this does not make sense. Sometime today, take a break, put on some music you love, and dance. Then return to your task with fresh energy and gratitude for your passion.

## AUGUST 11

*Being curious is a high state of being.*

LIVING YOUR YOGA: When you are curious, you're not sure you know, you're a little empty, and you're willing to learn. These qualities bring you into the present. And being present is at the heart of practicing yoga. What are you curious about today?

## AUGUST 12
*What do two-year-olds find so fun about mud puddles?*

LIVING YOUR YOGA: If you take a two-year-old on a walk after a rain, you know he likes to stop, look, and splash, in utter delight. Find some time today to become like that two-year-old, and find delight in the world, if only for a minute.


## AUGUST 13
*Movies are flickering pictures that appear to have form; so are my thoughts.*

LIVING YOUR YOGA: The greatest freedom in life is freedom from one's thoughts. Thoughts are just neurotransmitters locking into receptor sites: they are not the truth. Sit quietly for a few minutes whenever you can, and just watch the incessant rise and fall of thoughts. Let them go and wish them well, but don't believe them.


## AUGUST 14
*I can only be driven crazy by someone I truly love.*

LIVING YOUR YOGA: Attachment and aversion are first cousins. What I love and what I hate both control me. Today practice the pose you love most and the pose you hate most. Allow a space for equanimity to arise.

## AUGUST 15

*Wasted time is the time I spend not being present with my life.*

**LIVING YOUR YOGA:** There is really no such thing as wasted time if I am fully present with myself as each moment arises. Right now, stop, take a breath, observe what you are feeling, note what you are thinking, and look at what is going on around you. Hold these observations lightly and evenly. Practice this whenever you can, and the moment will not be wasted.

## AUGUST 16

*If you want to understand wonder, look at the face of a child closely examining a bug.*

**LIVING YOUR YOGA:** Losing touch with your wonder is sad. Wonder perfectly combines curiosity, gratitude, and presence. Today find something to observe in wonder: a flower, the sky, a tree, and notice how this reconnects you with life.

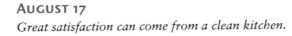

## AUGUST 17

*Great satisfaction can come from a clean kitchen.*

**LIVING YOUR YOGA:** We do not need fancy things to bring us joy. Choose a room or part of a room, and spend twenty minutes creating order there. Throw away what you can. Then enjoy the space and simplicity in this part of your world.

## AUGUST 18

*Which do you want: perfection or wholeness?*

**LIVING YOUR YOGA:** Often we strive for perfection. But perfection is unattainable, and striving for it limits us. Today sit quietly for a few minutes. As you breathe, imagine becoming a large container within which to hold your perfection and imperfection. When you can hold both, then you experience your wholeness.

## AUGUST 19

*Bend over backwards once a day.*

LIVING YOUR YOGA: Not only does a physical backbend strengthen your back and open your chest, but a mental backbend enriches your life. Today find an opportunity to stretch your mind by choosing something different and opening to a new experience. How did it go?

## AUGUST 20

*Who among us has the extra time to not live every moment fully?*

LIVING YOUR YOGA: What possibility does this moment hold? All possibilities. Without the clear awareness of this simple fact, life gets bogged down in unimportant things. Today choose as your Mantra of Daily Living: *This very moment.* Silently repeat this phrase whenever you remember it, and live it, too.

## AUGUST 21

*What is my intention for today?*

**LIVING YOUR YOGA:** Creating a clear intention for your day is powerful. This morning, choose a one-sentence intention for your day. It can be as simple as deciding to do one thing at a time or as grand as deciding to get married. Say your intention out loud in one simple sentence, and then follow it.

## AUGUST 22

*Practice the presence of God.*

**LIVING YOUR YOGA:** Treat everyone you meet today as an expression of the Divine. Then, before you sleep, reflect on how full of love you feel.

## AUGUST 23

*Yoga is not about touching your toes; it is about what you learn on the way down.*

**LIVING YOUR YOGA:** We tend to forget that asana is a process of self-discovery, not a bunch of exercises. Today when you practice, do every pose to only two-thirds of your ability. Focus on the experience, not the goal.


## AUGUST 24

*A short nap can make all the difference.*

**LIVING YOUR YOGA:** This afternoon, find a quiet place and lie down for twenty minutes. The rest of your day will be more enjoyable for you and those around you.


## AUGUST 25

*Ambivalence is part of every human relationship.*

**LIVING YOUR YOGA:** We all feel ambivalent, even about the most important people in our lives. When you have those feelings today, stop and take a deep breath, and let yourself be as ambivalent as possible. Then smile and go on with your day.

## AUGUST 26
*Everyone needs a pair of red shoes.*

**LIVING YOUR YOGA:** Sometimes practicality interferes with living fully. If you don't own a pair of red shoes, buy a pair and go dancing with someone you love as soon as possible!


## AUGUST 27
*A yoga class is a support group for people who can't do yoga.*

**LIVING YOUR YOGA:** Do you shrink from trying something because you judge yourself as not good enough? If so, remember that your yoga class is not full of experts; it is made up of *practitioners* of yoga. Go to class today, and practice from your heart.


## AUGUST 28
*The emotions of daily life are the stuff of our transformation.*

**LIVING YOUR YOGA:** Spend today observing your emotions: irritation, boredom, anxiety. Let them rise and fall and remember, you are not your feelings. They offer you insight into yourself, that's all. Let them go.

## AUGUST 29

*Excitement is the surface of fear.*

**LIVING YOUR YOGA:** Notice today what excites you. Then look deeper and see what it is about that exciting thing that stimulates fear in you. Notice how your excitement is tied to your fear.

## AUGUST 30

*I am a ship under full sail.*

**LIVING YOUR YOGA:** Stand up and spread your arms out wide. Take a deep breath and say aloud, *I am a ship under full sail.* Celebrate your power.

## AUGUST 31

*Center in your heart instead of your brain.*

**LIVING YOUR YOGA:** Sit quietly and let your awareness settle in the area of your heart. Stay here as you take and release ten breaths. Then come from this place as you go about the rest of your day.

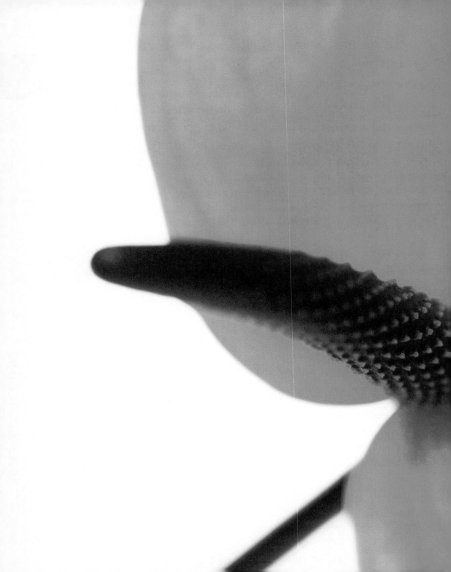

SEPTEMBER

## SEPTEMBER 1
*Listening heals a lot of grief and sadness.*

LIVING YOUR YOGA: Someone in your life needs to be heard, needs your attention. Today take the opportunity to listen to her for ten minutes, without planning your reply.

## SEPTEMBER 2
*If you want to be loving, first accept your ability to hate.*

LIVING YOUR YOGA: Love and hate are the opposite ends of a pendulum swing and are related through passion. To allow yourself to love fully, today resolve to accept your ability to hate. Do not act on that hate, but rather notice it is a part of you, and let compassion surround it.

## SEPTEMBER 3
*Everything you really need to know is in your own heart.*

LIVING YOUR YOGA: It is easy to get caught up in the belief that others know more than you do. True knowledge is more than just a collection of facts. Today trust yourself more, and live from that trust.

## SEPTEMBER 4

*Despair is anger turned inward.*

LIVING YOUR YOGA: Despair is an emotion built on thoughts. The next time you are feeling down about your life, ask yourself this question: *Am I feeling trapped, as if there is no choice in my situation right now?* Thinking you are stuck can stimulate and contribute to depression. Get up and go for a brisk fifteen-minute walk right now. Focus on the myriad choices life actually offers you.

## SEPTEMBER 5

*Tension is your body's response to the past.*

LIVING YOUR YOGA: Close your eyes and notice where you are holding tension in your body. This holding is related to your thoughts from the past. Find time today to lie in Savasana (Basic Relaxation Pose), supporting your head and under your knees, covering your eyes. Consciously observe your tension for fifteen minutes. Watch it melt away.

## SEPTEMBER 6

*Simplicity carried to extreme is elegance.*

LIVING YOUR YOGA: Choose an ordinary task, such as cutting an orange. Collect your tools and begin. Focus simply on one hand holding the orange, the movement of the knife through the fruit's skin, the sound as the knife strikes the chopping board. Notice the sunny brilliance of the orange flesh. Gather the pieces and put them in a bowl. Eat and taste.

## SEPTEMBER 7

*God has given us a delicious banana, and we are eating the peel.*

LIVING YOUR YOGA: Sit quietly and notice how many of your thoughts are about things that are truly unimportant in the scope of a whole life. Inhale, and as you exhale, focus on the gifts of life and the presence of someone to love. Then continue your day with a lighter heart.

## SEPTEMBER 8

*Wisdom is understanding the connection of all things;*
*enlightenment is being that connection.*

LIVING YOUR YOGA: Look at a shirt in your closet. Have you ever thought about how many people contributed to it hanging there? The shirt has in it the soil that grew the cotton, the sun and rain that nourished it, the people who picked it, those who spun it, those who wove it, and so much more. Before you put it on, offer silent gratitude for how we are all connected.

## SEPTEMBER 9

*Allow yourself to become a bigger container to hold all of life.*

LIVING YOUR YOGA: Sit quietly with a long spine and slightly dropped head. As you breathe, visualize your awareness expanding until is holds this whole moment as it is: sounds, sights, and smells. Take it all in and let it all go. Observe the storms we call thoughts, rising and falling. Remain for ten minutes, and then slowly get up to live your day fully.

## SEPTEMBER 10

*What seems like controlling your mind is only the dominance of one part of your mind over another part. Soon it will switch.*

LIVING YOUR YOGA: The mind cannot be controlled; it can be observed with love. When you step on your yoga mat today, come with curiosity. Notice how the mind first loves a pose, then is bored with it, then hates the pose. It keeps changing. Watch it with love.

## SEPTEMBER 11

*All security is false.*

LIVING YOUR YOGA: We spend lots of time in life trying to manipulate the things and people around us so we will feel safe. But nothing is secure, because all things change. Today notice how you cling to control as a strategy to feel safe. Instead, choose to embrace the absolute truth of change, and then notice how much safer you feel.

## SEPTEMBER 12

*Trying to be calm creates agitation; instead start with being present with your agitation.*

**LIVING YOUR YOGA:** The residue of effort is agitation, not calmness. Today on your yoga mat, find the calmness behind the agitation your thoughts create during asana. Attach yourself to this calmness.

## SEPTEMBER 13

*The secret to living well is never to do as much as you can.*

**LIVING YOUR YOGA:** Many of us measure our self-worth by how much we get accomplished each day. Consider this: our worth is not based on accomplishment but on our existence as a whole human being. Today resolve to do 10 percent less and enjoy yourself more.

## SEPTEMBER 14

*Because I am so rarely there, the most exotic place on Earth is where I am right now.*

LIVING YOUR YOGA: Where are you? Are you here right now? Close your eyes and listen. Then open them and look around. Whenever you can today, remember to be where you are.

## SEPTEMBER 15

*Letting go means realizing you weren't in charge anyway.*

LIVING YOUR YOGA: We often worry about so many things, most of them beyond our control. Just today, let go whenever you can by embracing the understanding that you are not in charge of the world.

## SEPTEMBER 16

*A white lie is any lie that you have decided it is okay to tell.*

**LIVING YOUR YOGA:** One of the basic teachings of yoga is to practice *satya,* or truth. Today when the urge to tell a white lie arises, counter it first with telling your truth to yourself, and then by telling your truth to others in a loving way.

## SEPTEMBER 17

*The body is as holy as the spirit.*

**LIVING YOUR YOGA:** Seeing the body and spirit as separate is a way of denigrating the temple that houses a treasure. Today choose to do something that nurtures your body in a way that you enjoy.

## SEPTEMBER 18

*More is not always the answer.*

**LIVING YOUR YOGA:** In this busy, busy world, we often believe that having a little more time is the answer. But you already have all the time there is in the Universe. Today do a little less, and let the spaciousness of time surround you.

## SEPTEMBER 19

*Which do you want: the pain of staying where you are, or the pain of growth?*

**LIVING YOUR YOGA:** We all want to avoid pain. But to be alive is to have pain of some kind. Some of this pain is self-created. Sit quietly today and consider an important choice you need to make. Ask yourself which pain you want—the pain of moving through your challenge, or the pain of avoiding it.

## SEPTEMBER 20

*Work for peace, but do it from a place of contentment.*

**LIVING YOUR YOGA:** We all want peace, both inner peace and peace in the world. Today chose one act of kindness to self or another, offered from a place of contentment, and you will create peace in that moment.

## SEPTEMBER 21
*What does this moment say?*

LIVING YOUR YOGA: When you get on your yoga mat, notice how your practice consists of telling your body what to do. Today when you practice, actively listen to what your body is telling you, and practice from that.


## SEPTEMBER 22
*The state of absorption is halfway to enlightenment.*

LIVING YOUR YOGA: Do you remember the absolute absorption you felt as a child when you were playing your favorite game? That level of focus is the first step of being fully realized. Today find something you love and focus on it completely for ten minutes—no judgments, no goals.

## SEPTEMBER 23

*The nature of the mind is to be agitated.*

**LIVING YOUR YOGA:** There is no such thing as a calm mind. Even during sleep, your mind is spinning. Practicing meditation therefore is the art of just being with your mental agitation, without the need to control or eliminate it. This process creates a disidentification with your thoughts that is the basis of all true freedom. Today sit quietly for ten minutes and watch the agitations we call mind.

## SEPTEMBER 24

*When you try to protect people by not telling them the truth, you multiply their suffering.*

**LIVING YOUR YOGA:** We think we're being loving to others by protecting them from the truth. But this creates the suffering of their learning not to trust us. Today make a commitment to tell the truth to those you love.

## SEPTEMBER 25

*Give up your attachment to the way you think things are, so you can experience things as they actually are.*

**LIVING YOUR YOGA:** Our beliefs create a screen between what is and how we want things to be. Yoga is a practice to help us let go of that screen and live authentically. What belief can you let go of today?

## SEPTEMBER 26

*Just for today, am I going to relive my past or create my present?*

**LIVING YOU YOGA:** How much time do you spend thinking about what might have been? Right now make a commitment to focus on this day, this asana, this moment.

## SEPTEMBER 27

*Fear is never about the present moment.*

**LIVING YOUR YOGA:** When one is in a truly life-threatening situation, there is often a sense of calmness more than anything. Today when you feel afraid, notice if you are truly present, and if not, then take a breath and drop down into your belly and into this moment.

## SEPTEMBER 28

*The yoga mat is my refuge.*

**LIVING YOUR YOGA:** What can I do today to make my yoga mat a place of deep refuge? Do I need to change its location or change the attitude that I bring to it?

## SEPTEMBER 29

*We spend most of our time* doing *instead of* being.

**LIVING YOUR YOGA:** Our culture honors accomplishment and action over being. Make sure you spend some time just being today. Find some time to hang out on the back porch, either literally or figuratively, and enjoy life.

## SEPTEMBER 30

*Embrace the confusion.*

**LIVING YOUR YOGA:** We tend to reject feeling confused. Today when you feel confused, take a deep breath, and as you exhale, drop down into your confusion and be the best confused person in the world. Don't let confusion interfere with your ability to be happy. It's just what is happening.

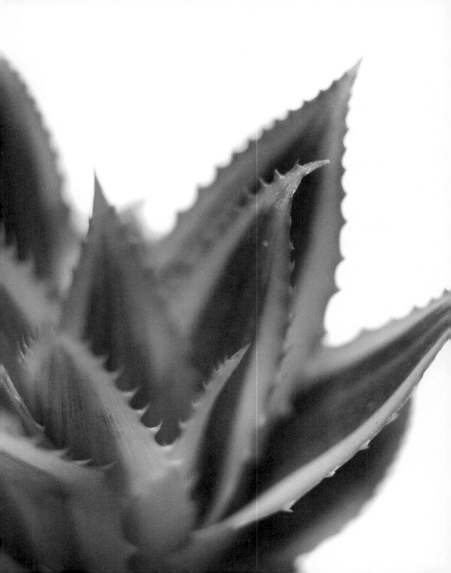

OCTOBER

## OCTOBER 1

*Slowing down is the same thing as waking up.*

**LIVING YOUR YOGA:** Find an ordinary task, like folding the laundry. Then do it today at a slow enough pace that you really notice it: the smell and warmth of the clothes, the colors and textures of the fabrics, and the order and satisfaction that arises from the neat pile. Now, try another task with that attitude. Your day will not only be productive but nourishing.

## OCTOBER 2

*Just being here, you are good enough.*

**LIVING YOUR YOGA:** Sit down, breathe, and remember that you are already complete and whole. Carry this awareness with you always.

## OCTOBER 3

*We bring the world our goodness.*

**LIVING YOUR YOGA:** Too often, we focus on our faults and shortcomings. Today remember that you can offer the world your best self.

## OCTOBER 4

*Busyness is our attempt to gain approval.*

**LIVING YOUR YOGA:** If you are addicted to being busy, sit down, collect yourself, and plan some time today, even if it is five minutes, in which there is no goal to accomplish other than simply being.

## OCTOBER 5

*Unless you take time to nurture yourself every single day, you can't give fully to others.*

**LIVING YOUR YOGA:** Taking care of others' needs cannot be done well and willingly without taking care of yourself. Plan a time to nurture yourself for at least twenty minutes today and for a whole day as soon as you can.

## OCTOBER 6

*The worse thing is to attempt to live someone else's life.*

**LIVING YOUR YOGA:** Sometimes someone else's life looks better than yours. Today find three things that you love about your life and celebrate them.

## OCTOBER 7

*Can you practice in a way that does not create violence to yourself?*

LIVING YOUR YOGA: Discipline is about consistency, not force. Today when you step on your yoga mat, notice any thoughts you may have about inflicting the poses on yourself. For a change, practice whatever you love with lightness. That lightness will become the residue left inside when your practice is over.


## OCTOBER 8

*Even if you can bend forward and place your palms flat on the floor, you are not guaranteed happiness.*

LIVING YOUR YOGA: Yoga practice is a strategy for being happy. The way it works, however, is a paradox. Yoga teaches us to discover the happiness that *already* lives within us. Touching your toes does not create happiness; it slows you down enough to experience it. Remember this today when you practice your poses.

## OCTOBER 9
*Harmony is the beginning, not the goal.*

**LIVING YOUR YOGA:** Practice a twenty-minute Savasana (Basic Relaxation Pose) and notice how you feel at the end. This sense of harmony is not the point of practice but the *foundation* of practice for all the interactions with self and others today.

## OCTOBER 10
*The way you move reveals the way you think.*

**LIVING YOUR YOGA:** How do you approach your asana practice? Are your movements exploratory and loving or harsh and demanding? Today when you practice asana, notice the quality of your movements.

## OCTOBER 11
*God has all points of view at once.*

**LIVING YOUR YOGA:** Today when you are attached to your point of view as better than someone else's, remember the bigger picture.

## OCTOBER 12

*The two most important poses are standing up with awareness and lying down for deep relaxation.*

**LIVING YOUR YOGA:** Step on your yoga mat and begin with Tadasana (Mountain Pose). Root your feet downward and open your heart to the heavens. Finish your practice with a twenty-minute Savasana (Basic Relaxation Pose). Standing well relieves the body, and relaxing deeply relieves the mind.

## OCTOBER 13

*How you talk to yourself matters.*

**LIVING YOUR YOGA:** Our beliefs create a filter through which we see the world. To become free of their power, today pay attention to what you say. Instead of saying *I can't*, say *I'm having difficulty right now.* This will create a space between the present and your beliefs about the present.

## OCTOBER 14
*We are attached to difficulties.*

**LIVING YOUR YOGA:** Our tendency is to focus on what is wrong with a pose. What can you celebrate in this pose today?

## OCTOBER 15
*Who do you blame for your problems?*

**LIVING YOUR YOGA:** Problems arise. Today remember there is a difference between blaming yourself for problems and taking responsibility for them.

## OCTOBER 16
*It's about learning, not about getting it right.*

**LIVING YOUR YOGA:** Remember today that learning is not something we stop doing when we leave school. Learning is all there is. Realizing that your life is about learning will reduce self-judgment and contribute to your happiness.

## OCTOBER 17
*All we need to do is slow down.*

**LIVING YOUR YOGA:** Drive the speed limit.


## OCTOBER 18
*God hides wisdom in plain view.*

**LIVING YOUR YOGA:** If you look closely and listen attentively, you will see the wisdom in the slow stretch of a cat, in the persistent grass growing through the cracks in the sidewalk, in the cool beauty of the moon, and in the sound of your friend's voice. Celebrate them.


## OCTOBER 19
*Acceptance is seeing clearly what is.*

**LIVING YOUR YOGA:** Acceptance does not mean that we are necessarily happy with the way things are, but that we see the way things are. Today pick one circumstance in your life and be willing to see it the way it is. Just so.

## OCTOBER 20

*The most powerful things are unseen.*

**LIVING YOUR YOGA:** The unseen atom holds tremendous power. There is also power in other unseen things: love, friendship, forgiveness. Today remember to trust the power of the unseen.


## OCTOBER 21

*Ease is action without effort.*

**LIVING YOUR YOGA:** Ease does not mean doing nothing. Rather, it means that what you do flows from your core and does not require effort. What takes effort in your life? How can you find the ease in that activity today?

## OCTOBER 22

*The greatest avoidance strategy is* I don't have time.

LIVING YOUR YOGA: Everyone has the same amount of time every day. Resolve to make choices today that allow you to feel more spacious about time in your life.


## OCTOBER 23

*To practice yoga is to move out of our habits.*

LIVING YOUR YOGA: Stretching in asana is placing the body in a new and slightly unfamiliar position. Make a choice today that places you in an unfamiliar emotional or mental position, and watch the fun.


## OCTOBER 24

*No one comes to yoga unless they already know.*

LIVING YOUR YOGA: We may think that yoga practice will give us the answers to life. Today remember that you practice not to have the answers, but because you already have the answers in your heart.

## OCTOBER 25

*Forget enlightenment. Go for happiness.*

**LIVING YOUR YOGA:** Happiness is your birthright. Use your practice today to uncover the happiness of this very moment.


## OCTOBER 26

*All conflict springs from the false perception of duality.*

**LIVING YOUR YOGA:** You can only fight with someone if you see her as separate from you. Today remember that the belief in separation is the root of all suffering. Choose to see the other's point of view. No one is really separate from you.


## OCTOBER 27

*Relationship is the fundamental truth of the Universe.*

**LIVING YOUR YOGA:** Everything exists in relationship to everything else. Nothing exists alone. Therefore, all your choices and actions are part of the whole. Today choose words and actions that honor your relationship to nature and self.

## OCTOBER 28
*If you think you like a yoga pose, hold it for five minutes.*

**LIVING YOUR YOGA:** The mind jumps back and forth between like and dislike. Select a yoga pose you think you like, and see what the mind tells you about it after you have held it for five minutes. And this is the mind we trust!

## OCTOBER 29
*Breathe in life through your cells.*

**LIVING YOUR YOGA:** Lie on your yoga mat with your chest and head slightly elevated; place a roll under your knees, with your arms comfortably out to the sides. Take ten long inhalations and ten long exhalations. When you do so, take in life completely as you inhale, and let go into life as you exhale. Try this breathing technique today when you feel bored, or disconnected, or afraid.

## OCTOBER 30
*Yoga is a practice of observation and faith.*

**LIVING YOUR YOGA:** When you practice your asana today, have faith that you know what to do and how to do it. Observe your thoughts as they arise, without judging them.

## OCTOBER 31
*Your body is not the problem.*

**LIVING YOUR YOGA:** Not able to bend backward? Can't touch your toes? As you step on your mat today, remember that your body is not a problem to be overcome. Instead, enjoy what you can do right now, and do it with love.

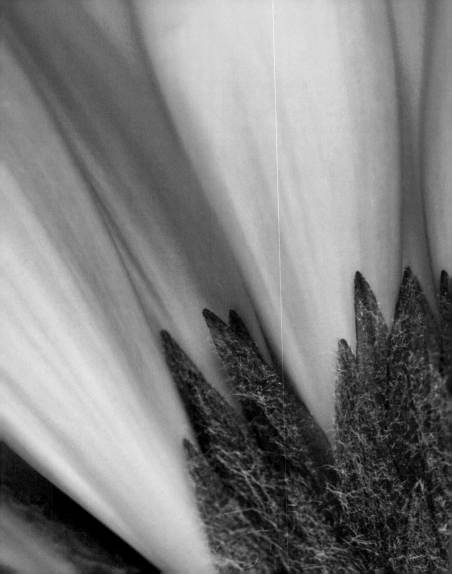

NOVEMBER

## NOVEMBER 1
*Don't confuse ambition with discipline.*

**LIVING YOUR YOGA:** Discipline is not supported by ambition but by consistency. When you practice yoga today, focus on consistency and not on forcing yourself to do more, just for the sake of your ego.

## NOVEMBER 2
*Yoga is not only about stretching your muscles, but also about the residue of awareness that comes afterward.*

**LIVING YOUR YOGA:** The pose is not the yoga; yoga is the inner state the pose creates. Pay more attention today to the state that is created by your poses.

## NOVEMBER 3
*Everything everyone says to you is a request.*

**LIVING YOUR YOGA:** To improve your communication today, translate whatever anyone says to you as a request for attention and respect. The words they say don't matter; hear the deeper words spoken from their hearts.

## NOVEMBER 4

*Let your heart yearn for heaven, but keep your brain focused on the here and now.*

LIVING YOUR YOGA: Stand in Tadasana (Mountain Pose). Focus on moving your heart gently upward and your brain gently downward. Notice how centered you feel. Practice this whenever you can today.

## NOVEMBER 5

*Teach for yourself; practice for your students.*

LIVING YOUR YOGA: Do not be afraid to teach what comes from your heart today. And when you practice your own yoga, focus instead on what you can learn to teach others.

## NOVEMBER 6

*We only see what we believe.*

LIVING YOUR YOGA: We think that we believe what we see. Actually, the opposite is true: we begin with belief, and then we see. What do you believe in today? Yourself?

## NOVEMBER 7

*Emotions arise when beliefs are challenged.*

LIVING YOUR YOGA: Today notice when you are agitated, or angry, or upset. Then ask yourself: *What belief of mine has just been challenged?*

## NOVEMBER 8

*There is no place that is not your yoga mat.*

LIVING YOUR YOGA: Practicing yoga need not be confined to your mat. Imagine today that the whole world is your yoga mat and everything that happens to you is an asana. Remember to breathe.

## NOVEMBER 9

*Practice is an intention, not a location.*

LIVING YOUR YOGA: Step on your mat today and create a practice intention with a Mantra for Daily Living, such as *I will breathe with awareness,* or *I will remain present in my belly.* Then carry this intention into the rest of your day.

## NOVEMBER 10

*The most radical thing we can do is to be deeply present.*

**LIVING YOUR YOGA:** We all want to change the world for the better. The best way to do it is to do practices like asana and meditation that help us to be present. When we are present, we are more likely to make choices that support peace and harmony. Practice today with this in mind.

## NOVEMBER 11

*If you act from your beliefs, you think you know reality before you actually perceive it.*

**LIVING YOUR YOGA:** What we think about the world is not the world: it is only our thoughts. Sit quietly today for ten minutes and watch your thoughts become beliefs and then dissolve again into thoughts.

## November 12

*The mind can only plan the future from its experience of the past.*

LIVING YOUR YOGA: Scientists tell us that when we think we are planning for the future, we are actually basing those thoughts on past experience. Without a past, we cannot conceive of a future. Practice today with the intention of being present with the sensations of the moment and not your thoughts about them.

## November 13

*The ability to understand the cost of my choices before I make them is the beginning of wisdom.*

LIVING YOUR YOGA: Whatever choice you make, that choice affects the world in ways you will never know. When you make choices today, make them with love.

## NOVEMBER 14

*Contentment is a choice I can make every day.*

**LIVING YOUR YOGA:** The Yoga Sutra instructs us to actively practice *santosa,* or contentment. Can you actively practice contentment with your asana practice today?

## NOVEMBER 15

*Asana is a mental practice that expresses itself through the body.*

**LIVING YOUR YOGA:** No one really understands the relationship of the mind and the body, of the physical and the mental, of thought and action. When you practice your asana today, do so with your whole body and whole mind.

## NOVEMBER 16

*God is looking for you.*

**LIVING YOUR YOGA:** Our practice is often based on the belief that we need to focus on seeking health, seeking wholeness, seeking God. Today as you practice asana, pranayama, and meditation, remember that God is also seeking you. Open your heart and receive the Divine.

## NOVEMBER 17

*An adult is a human being who believes she should do something perfectly the first time she tries.*

LIVING YOUR YOGA: Watch a child learn to walk, and you will be instructed in the power of persistence as she falls down and gets up, time and again. As adults, we become impatient or discouraged when we can't learn a new skill on our first try. Today when you practice, allow yourself to fail. Remember, it is called *yoga practice* not *yoga performance*.

## NOVEMBER 18

*Kindness is gratitude in action.*

LIVING YOUR YOGA: What one person, circumstance, or thing are you grateful for today? Express your gratitude quietly to yourself, and then live your gratitude by offering kindness to those you meet throughout the day.

## NOVEMBER 19

*Compassion begins in my heart and ends in the heart of the other.*

**LIVING YOUR YOGA:** Sometimes we believe that compassion for others is more important than compassion for self. In reality, they are inseparable. When you practice today, hold yourself in a compassionate embrace.

## NOVEMBER 20

*A bowl of soup lovingly made can cure many ills.*

**LIVING YOUR YOGA:** Sometimes the simplest things give us the most profound comfort. Make some soup today and enjoy its delicious warmth with gratitude.

## NOVEMBER 21

Saucha, *or purity, is not a measure of my actions and their results, but a measure of my intention.*

**LIVING YOUR YOGA:** What intention guides your work today?

## NOVEMBER 22

*You cannot be a whole and healthy person unless you are whole and healthy in your sexuality.*

**LIVING YOUR YOGA:** Your sexuality is life expressing itself through you. Trust it and live it with compassion, honesty, and respect today.

## NOVEMBER 23

*To practice yoga is to open up to our physical, mental, and emotional difficulties and limitations, whether that is a tight hamstring or a wounded psyche.*

**LIVING YOUR YOGA:** What we call our difficulties are often just the thoughts we have about our situation. Today remember that your difficulties are just chances to let go, so do it.

## NOVEMBER 24

*To practice yoga is to know the Self; to know the Self is to know God; to know God is to be free.*

**LIVING YOUR YOGA:** The practice of yoga is not about anything else but freedom. Practice your poses and your meditation today with this in mind, and do not get caught up in some external measure of success.

## NOVEMBER 25

*Ahimsa, or nonharming, is the first practice.*

**LIVING YOUR YOGA:** Without ahimsa, all practice is violence. As you step on your yoga mat, lovingly accept yourself as you are, and then let your practice emerge from here. Acceptance can never come from violence to self.

## NOVEMBER 26

*Anytime you are present in the moment and deeply enjoying yourself is a meditative moment.*

**LIVING YOUR YOGA:** How often are you distracted from whatever you are doing? Take advantage of today by finding something that absorbs you and offers you enjoyment at the same time.

## NOVEMBER 27

*Schedule yourself a "pajama day" once a week.*

**LIVING YOUR YOGA:** We are so busy, busy, busy. Every week, plan ahead for a day or part of a day when you can stay home and rest or do simple tasks. Resting is part of life, too.

## NOVEMBER 28

*Where can you go that God isn't?*

**LIVING YOUR YOGA:** Everything that exists has aliveness in it. Today celebrate the Consciousness that pervades all people and all things.

## NOVEMBER 29

*I can't be both grateful and greedy at the same time.*

**LIVING YOUR YOGA:** Today when you feel that others have more than you and you are missing something, name ten things that you are grateful for.

## NOVEMBER 30

*Enjoyment feeds my soul.*

**LIVING YOUR YOGA:** Think of the joy you experienced as a child. Today make a promise to yourself that you will slow down and enjoy something beautiful, just because it exists.

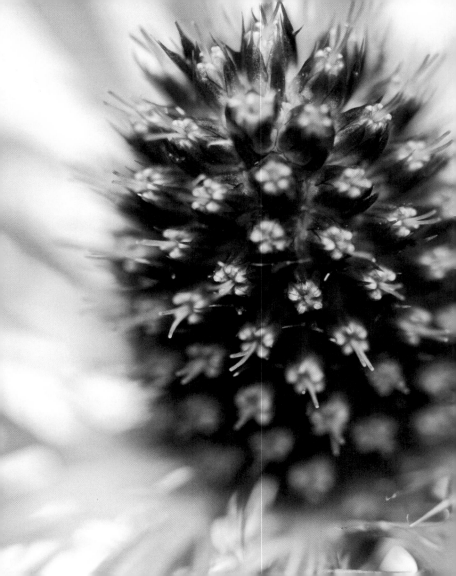

DECEMBER

## DECEMBER 1

*Find your natural rhythm; honor the natural rhythm of others.*

**LIVING YOUR YOGA:** We feel happier when we move with our body's own rhythms. Find a day soon, stay home, and find out what your natural rhythms are. For example, eat when you are hungry, sleep when you are tired. Honor your tempo.

## DECEMBER 2

*Be twice as clear about money with your friends as with others.*

**LIVING YOUR YOGA:** Money is just a form of energy, but it has different meanings for each of us. Today make a commitment that you will be very clear in all your money dealings with friends, so as to honor your precious friendship and keep it open.

## DECEMBER 3

*Spend five minutes every morning reconnecting*
*with the Sacred.*

**LIVING YOUR YOGA:** What is Sacred for you? This morning, spend five minutes quietly reflecting on whatever it is, and then carry that awareness with you throughout the day.

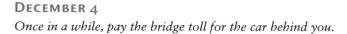

## DECEMBER 4

*Once in a while, pay the bridge toll for the car behind you.*

LIVING YOUR YOGA: Today do something nice for a complete stranger. Enjoy watching their surprise.

## DECEMBER 5

*No one has the answers to life; everyone is the answer to life.*

LIVING YOUR YOGA: Even the most brilliant among us cannot explain the most important questions: Why are we here? What is our purpose? What happens after we die? Remember today that just being fully you is enough.

## DECEMBER 6

*Remember to give your attention to what is worthy of it.*

LIVING YOUR YOGA: If you care about nothing, your life will be lonely. If you care about everything, you will live in a perpetual state of upset. Just for today, can you find the perfect balance between involvement and detachment?

## DECEMBER 7
*If you are going to worry, enjoy it completely.*

**LIVING YOUR YOGA:** Worrying is focusing on the future; it takes you away from what is. But if you like it, do it completely! This will make you smile, and you will probably stop worrying about what you can't control. Make today a day of conscious worrying.

## DECEMBER 8
*Once in your life, eat a brownie for breakfast.*

**LIVING YOUR YOGA:** Sometimes doing something whimsical feeds the soul and lightens our life. Find something whimsical to do today and enjoy it.

## DECEMBER 9
*Everything is a miracle.*

**LIVING YOUR YOGA:** When you lose your wonder, life loses its juice. Look around you today and notice the simple miracles you see: babies, the sun, birds, the stars. Keep a sense of wonder with you all day.

## DECEMBER 10

*Now.*

**LIVING YOUR YOGA:** Whenever you can today, come back to this very moment. Do this by paying attention to your breath.

## DECEMBER 11

*Love is what arises in me when I sense the Divine in the other.*

**LIVING YOUR YOGA:** When you feel loving feelings, you are connected to the Divine. What stimulates loving feelings in you right now?

## DECEMBER 12

*All longing is the longing for God.*

**LIVING YOUR YOGA:** We all long for acceptance and wholeness. Sit quietly and feel your longing. Know that the cessation of longing comes from your connection to Divinity. Find a way to strengthen that connection today.

### DECEMBER 13
*Cultivating empathy for myself will change the world.*

LIVING YOUR YOGA: Hold yourself gently today, offer yourself empathy, and you will create a space inside for compassion to arise. When compassion arises, act from that space.

### DECEMBER 14
*Everyone is your teacher.*

LIVING YOUR YOGA: The person ahead of you in traffic is not a nuisance; he is your teacher and is teaching you patience. Commit to seeing everyone as your teacher throughout the day, and you will feel happier and more content.

### DECEMBER 15
*Reality doesn't exist.*

LIVING YOUR YOGA: Each of us has our own view of reality. Remember this when you are convinced you are right: right about the government, right about what your neighbors should do, right about how an asana should be practiced.

## DECEMBER 16
*The ability to laugh at myself is a measure of my mental health.*

**LIVING YOUR YOGA:** Life presents challenges. Even so, find something funny about yourself to laugh at today.

## DECEMBER 17
*Perspective is the beginning of freedom.*

**LIVING YOUR YOGA:** So much of our suffering is caused by the lack of perspective. Think of an argument you had recently. Take out a piece of paper and write down the argument from the other person's point of view. Hold as precious this new perspective.

## DECEMBER 18
*No one is right.*

**LIVING YOUR YOGA:** If you focus on being right, you can only see the other person as wrong. This form of thinking creates division. Today focus on being right for yourself right now, instead of being right over everyone all the time. This will bring connection and mutuality to your relationships.

## DECEMBER 19

*When I move at the speed of my body and not the speed of my brain, I am happier.*

LIVING YOUR YOGA: Today on your yoga mat, spend more time listening to your body and moving at its speed, and less time telling your body what to do and making it move at the speed of your thoughts.

## DECEMBER 20

*Choose contentment.*

LIVING YOUR YOGA: In this very moment, you can chose contentment—and in the next, and in the next, and in the next.

## DECEMBER 21

*The changing seasons show us the absolute reliability of change.*

LIVING YOUR YOGA: Nothing is more dependable than change. Look at the moon in the night sky, and make a date with yourself to look at it each night for the coming week. Take comfort in the changes.

## DECEMBER 22

*I can only call someone an enemy if I am disconnected
from myself.*

**LIVING YOUR YOGA:** Believing someone is my enemy means I have
not yet seen her suffering. Sit quietly and think about someone you
consider an enemy. Now imagine the suffering that person is experiencing. Inhale, and as you exhale, let go of your enemy images.

## DECEMBER 23

*What are they going to put on your tombstone? We miss her
so much; her hamstrings were so loose.*

**LIVING YOUR YOGA:** The ability to perform advanced asana only
means that you have the ability to perform advanced asana. Today
when you practice asana, no matter how advanced a practitioner
you are, do only very simple poses. Remember, asana is only a part
of yoga.

## DECEMBER 24
*If you want to understand one of the great mysteries of life, bake a loaf of bread from scratch.*

LIVING YOUR YOGA: Create some time today to bake a loaf of bread. Celebrate the growth of the yeast and drink in the smell as the bread bakes. When it is done, eat a piece in gratitude.


## DECEMBER 25
*Get over yourself.*

LIVING YOUR YOGA: We often spend our days enmeshed in our own dramas. This is mildly interesting but ultimately boring. Remember today to say to yourself the ultimate Mantra for Daily Living: *Get over yourself.*


## DECEMBER 26
*There is no right or wrong, only opinion.*

LIVING YOUR YOGA: Scientists tell us that electrons have a "tendency" to exist. Maybe even electrons are an opinion. Then why argue about anything today?

## DECEMBER 27

*A healthy ego is not the problem; attachment to what ego wants is the problem.*

LIVING YOUR YOGA: Spend a few minutes today contemplating the difference between ego and egoism. A healthy ego creates your ability to have clear boundaries; egoism is an unhealthy attachment to having it your way all the time.

## DECEMBER 28

*Sit still every day.*

LIVING YOUR YOGA: Our lives are in motion, both mental and physical. Right now is the best moment to sit still and be. Sit still whenever you can today, even if only for a few minutes.

## DECEMBER 29

*Renunciation is an inner practice that is unrelated to how much I actually have.*

LIVING YOUR YOGA: What physical possessions do you really need? Today can you use your possessions, treat them with respect, and simultaneously not cling to them?

### DECEMBER 30
*Perfect technique in asana will not create happiness.*

**LIVING YOUR YOGA:** Happiness is not related to an achievement or any other external. Today allow yourself to be happy in the midst of whatever is happening around you, as imperfect as it may feel.

### DECEMBER 31
*Laugh!*

**LIVING YOUR YOGA:** Make a commitment today to laugh. Not only does it relax the diaphragm, but also connects us with ourselves and with others.

# ABOUT THE AUTHOR

JUDITH HANSON LASATER has taught yoga since 1971. She holds a doctorate in East–West psychology and is a physical therapist. She is president of the California Yoga Teachers Association, and serves on the advisory boards of *Yoga Journal* and *Healing Lifestyles*.

Her yoga training includes study with B. K. S. Iyengar in India and the United States. She teaches yoga classes and trains yoga teachers in kinesiology, yoga therapeutics, and the Yoga Sutra in the San Francisco Bay Area. She also gives workshops throughout the United States, and has taught in Australia, Bolivia, Canada, England, France, Indonesia, Japan, Mexico, Peru, and Russia.

She writes extensively on the therapeutic aspects of yoga. She is the author of:

- *Relax and Renew* (1995)
- *Living Your Yoga* (2000)
- *30 Essential Yoga Poses* (2003)
- *Yoga for Pregnancy* (2004)

- *Yoga Abs* (2005)
- *A Year of Living Your Yoga* (2006)

These books are published by Rodmell Press.

Her popular "Asana" column ran in *Yoga Journal* for thirteen years, and she continues to contribute articles on a variety of subjects. In addition, her writing has appeared in numerous magazines and books, including *Healing Lifestyles, Yoga International, Yoga Chicago, Ascent, LA Yoga, Natural Health, Sports Illustrated for Women, Prevention, Alternative Therapies, Numedx, International Journal of Yoga Therapy, Complementary Therapies in Rehabilitation, Yogini, The Woman's Book of Yoga and Health, Living Yoga, American Yoga, The New Yoga for People Over 50,* and *Lilias, Yoga, and Your Life.*

Judith Hanson Lasater lives in the San Francisco Bay Area with her family.

## Studying Yoga with Judith Hanson Lasater, Ph.D., P.T.

Judith Hanson Lasater offers ongoing yoga classes, leads yoga vacations, lectures and teaches at yoga conferences, and gives workshops and seminars, including Relax and Renew Seminars® and Living Your Yoga Seminars®. All are open to interested individuals, yoga teachers, and health care professionals. For her teaching schedule, visit:

- www.judithlasater.com
- www.restorativeyogateachers.com

In addition, Judith teaches a series of Tele-Classes, which are 60-minute, live, interactive training classes that are conducted over the telephone, through state-of-the-art teleconferencing bridge systems. She shares information, tools, and techniques to enhance students' lives, teaching, and personal practice. For more information, visit Yoga Spirit at www.yogaspirit.ca.

# FROM THE PUBLISHER

RODMELL PRESS publishes books on yoga, Buddhism, aikido, and Taoism. In the Bhagavadgita it is written, "Yoga is skill in action." It is our hope that our books will help individuals develop a more skillful practice—one that brings peace to their daily lives and to the earth.

We thank those whose support, encouragement, and practical advise sustain us in our efforts. In particular, we are grateful to Reb Anderson, B. K. S. Iyengar, Wendy Palmer, and Yvonne Rand for their inspiration.

To request a catalog or receive e-announcements about new titles, contact us at:

    (510) 841-3123 or (800) 841-3123    info@rodmellpress.com
    (510) 841-3123 (fax)    www.rodmellpress.com

Rodmell Press is distributed to the trade by Publishers Group West:

    (800) 788-3123    info@pgw.com
    (510) 528-5511 (sales fax)